The Internet for Surgeons

Springer

New York
Berlin
Heidelberg
Barcelona
Hong Kong
London
Milan
Paris
Singapore
Tokyo

THE
INTERNET
FOR
SURGEONS

with 40 Illustrations

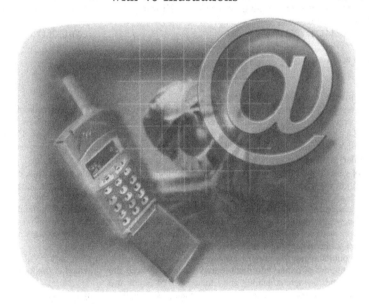

JEFF W. ALLEN, MD
University of Louisville School of Medicine
Louisville, Kentucky
USA

Foreword by Professor Sir Alfred Cuschieri, MD, and Hiram C. Polk, Jr., MD

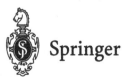 Springer

includes
CD-ROM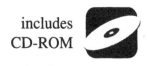

Jeff W. Allen, MD
Department of Surgery
University of Louisville School of Medicine
Louisville, KY 40252
USA

Library of Congress Cataloging-in-Publication Data
Allen, Jeffrey W. (Jeffrey Wayne), 1968–
    The Internet for surgeons / Jeffrey W. Allen.
      p. ; cm.
    Includes bibliographical references and index.
    ISBN 0-387-95319-1 (s/c : alk. paper)
    1. Surgery—Computer network resources. 2. Internet. 3. Surgeons. I. Title.
    [DNLM: 1. Internet. 2. Surgery. W 26.5 A427i 2001]
    RD31.5 .A35 2001
    004.67′8′0246171—dc21   2001032811

Printed on acid-free paper.

Production managed by Lesley Poliner; manufacturing supervised by Jeffrey Taub.
Typeset by Matrix Publishing Services, York, PA.
Printed and bound by Maple-Vail Book Manufacturing Group, York, PA.
Printed in the United States of America.

9 8 7 6 5 4 3 2 1

ISBN 0-387-95319-1   SPIN 10841725

Springer-Verlag   New York Berlin Heidelberg
A member of BertelsmannSpringer Science + Business Media GmbH

Foreword

Advances in surgery have reached an exponential scale, and the changes of the last decade of the twentieth century have become common practice. Imagination and foresight are the more visible standards for professional appointments than ever before. The fiber optic cable, computer, and Internet are the workhorses of this sea-change, and surgeons must master all of them to remain intellectually and technically up-to-date. There can be no better explanation for the genuine need for this book.

The transmission of knowledge and technical skills from one generation to another has been a common practice in surgery for nearly 200 years. Past experiences of surgeons have focused upon an understanding of disease states, a prompt diagnosis of a correctable illness and its appropriate evaluation, and most importantly, the technical conduct of an operation, where indicated, to provide relief to and/or cure of the patient. Fascinatingly, this little book tends to fulfill that same role with respect to the newly emerged technology of the Internet, computation, and telemedicine. In essence, this book seeks, and to a remarkable degree, achieves the transmission of both knowledge and technical skill in an easily usable and clearly written format.

Jeff W. Allen has provided an educational orientation with which he is familiar, both as a recent pupil and now as a teacher of surgical procedures. This is not unlike the kind of education that has gone on between trainee surgeons and master surgeons around the world. In this case, Dr. Allen serves as the Webmaster for the surgeon who wants to understand and use the Internet in a meaningful way.

There are few manuals or monographs that are easily readable, reasonably illustrated, and appropriately applicable to the world of the computer and the Internet itself. This handbook accomplishes that in a simple, readable fashion, with a variety of steps that can be easily followed. Contrary to the previous analogy here is a situation in which a younger surgeon is to some degree more likely to be teaching older surgeons about the extent and utilization of the Internet itself. This book is simple without being simplistic, and touches on virtually all of the entry-level bases necessary to productively use the Internet. There are both readily understood illustrations, examples and some frank and no-holds-barred advice about common mistakes that doctors can, and do, make with the Internet.

One of the most enjoyable components of the manual is the familiarization in step-wise fashion with both the lingo and the language of the Internet and its users. There is especially good insight into the surgical use of the Internet, which includes the ethical journals, which are now more and more promptly available on the Internet, and especially the growing capability of continuing medical education in both a convenient and inexpensive format.

The entire issue of the relationship with the patient is influenced by the computer. The doctor's personal Web page is a powerful dimension of this activity, fraught with great opportunities for misunderstanding as well as advanced education as is illustrated in the wryly-humorous examples of surgeons' communications with patients postoperatively. Less dependent on the geographic location in the United States than in the recent past, a high proportion of patients discuss an elective operation with a substantial amount of education and insight already gleaned by their sorties into the Internet. More often than not, we personally have found these prior inquiries productive and helpful as well as advancing and facilitating discussion. As always, it is probably worthwhile to document this kind of exchange or reference in the patient's formal record or chart.

The issue of robotic, remote, and telementored surgery is something that must be refined with the best effort to provide quality care to the patient in each and every step. It is obvious that such activities will occur and will grow in frequency. It is an ethical challenge, however, for the surgeon to be certain that this is a proper course as, for example, opposed to traditional referral bases for patients to individuals who are known to be skilled and experienced in a given procedure.

There is also a broad listing of some major industries, which impact on the surgical profession and for which there are appropriate references to their largely ethical and sensible purveying of both new and old products. The longtime guise not to be the first to try new things nor the last to lay old aside no doubt applies as much here as ever.

This manual represents a soup-to-nuts survey of the world of surgery, and the Internet as it exists in the very early years of the twenty-first century. No doubt, this will grow enormously. But, similarly, we believe that this handbook will be a benchmark by which others are measured and one that will provide safe, non-frustrating, and enjoyable access to a vast new dimension of surgical life.

Professor Sir Alfred Cuschieri
Department of Surgery and
   Molecular Oncology
University of Dundee
Dundee, Scotland

Hiram C. Polk, Jr., MD
Ben A. Reid Professor
   and Chairman
Department of Surgery
University of Louisville
Louisville, Kentucky

Series Preface

The Internet is the ultimate amalgamation of the Information Age and the Communication Age. It is a technology that took 40 years to become an overnight sensation, moving from the province of computer geeks to household utility in short order, once it was discovered. We have gone from thinking a URL was a form of alien presence to viewing it as a natural footnote to bus advertising.

Like the Internet itself, interest in computing, both local and distant, has grown exponentially. Now grandmothers send e-mails to their stockbrokers, meals are planned and the groceries purchased across the Web, and music videos can be previewed or concert tickets purchased—all with the help of the Internet. When our children come home from school, they are as likely to sign on to the Internet as they are to turn on the television. The Internet is a universal commodity, for those with access.

The American Internet User Survey found that more than 41.5 million adults in the United States actively are using the Internet. Of these Web users, 51% use the Web on a daily basis. It seems everybody needs to be connected to the Web, just as they all seem to need to make cell-phone calls while changing lanes in heavy traffic. The Internet is nothing less than a library card to the world. At the most basic level, the Internet is a high-speed web of worldwide computer-based information resources. It is a network of computer networks. One moment you can be browsing through the Library of Congress or looking at pictures from the National Library of Medicine, and the next moment conversing with a colleague in Indonesia.

What about the Internet and medicine? Well, we, physicians, sell information. That is what we do in medicine. That is what we always have done. Today, the difference is that we do it in an age built on information. Information, medical and otherwise, is all around us. From pocket pagers that deliver stock quotes and sports scores to palm-top digital assistance that wirelessly connects to the Internet, information is achieving the status of Oxygen[†]—it is all around us and invisible. Today, informa-

---

[†]Oxygen also is the name of a computing project at the Massachusetts Institute of Technology that is aimed at achieving this goal.

tion is managed, moved, and organized in ways never thought of in the past and will soon be managed in ways not yet conceived. In medicine, information is vital, but the exponential growth of knowledge available requires new approaches to its dissemination, access, and use. Central to this is the Internet. Information is now the province of anyone with a computer. This has led to "disintermediation": the ability of consumers to go directly to the source of information (or goods and services), bypassing the intermediate steps of providers. In medicine, this means that physicians obtain and distribute information in new ways, patients obtain and receive their information in new ways, and, together, patients and providers interact in new ways. Very little has remained the same, yet, fundamentally, nothing is different—we still sell information. Medicine has frequently led the way with new technology: We used print materials when books were in their infancy, we embraced the telephone like few other professions, pagers, two-way radio, and teleconferencing (telemedicine) were all adopted by medicine early in their development. The need for information always has driven this adoption, and it is no different for the Internet.

This series of texts on the Internet in medicine and in medical subspecialty areas hopes to assist in this natural evolution in two ways. First, it will help us understand the abilities of the Internet and know its tools so that we may capitalize on what the Internet holds for ourselves as physicians and for our patients. Secondly, the medical applications of the Internet have grown too rapidly and are too specialty-specific to explore in-depth in any single volume. Hence, the birth of specialty-specific volumes. When the first edition of *The Internet for Physicians* was published, it was mainly the technophile fringe that was surfing. The first edition attempted to introduce the concept of information transfer and communication and point the way toward a tool of the future. The second edition attempted to assuage trepidation in the use of this emerging tool and suggest the why and wherefore of being connected. The needs that drove those goals almost have completely disappeared. The third edition is more focussed on the medical aspects of the Internet and its use, and much less on the nuts and bolts of connecting and communicating through the Web. This evolution has opened the possibility of a series dedicated to the Internet in various specialties of medicine. Each of these volumes deals with specialty-specific aspects of the Internet, going beyond the general scope of *The Internet for Physicians*. Each author has been chosen for his or her expertise in medical computing, and they are each a recognized leader in their field. Each volume builds on fundamentals introduced in *The Internet for Physicians*. While each volume stands alone, they have all been created so that each fits within the same concept. As authors, we hope that this series will open new and exciting options for this new age of medical information. Surfs up!

Roger P. Smith, MD
University of Missouri–Kansas City School of Medicine
Kansas City, Missouri, USA
Author of *The Internet for Physicians*

Preface

During a recent meeting of the Society of American Gastrointestinal Endoscopic Surgeons (SAGES) in my hometown of Louisville, Kentucky, the following statement was made: "The revolution in surgery already has occurred. All that is left now is the evolution." Although the speaker at the SAGES meeting was referring to the laparoscopic method of operating, the same thing can now be said of the Internet.

The revolution of the World Wide Web and electronic mail happened, for the most part, in the early 1990s. Today, our use, as physicians, of Internet technologies continues to evolve. I hope that this book will help you evolve into an Internet savvy surgeon. Most patients today will enter a doctor's office with more knowledge about their condition than the patients of 20 or 30 years ago. Arguably, this is a good thing. The source of their information often is one or more World Wide Web pages about their diagnosis. I hope this book prepares you to deal with this situation, knowing that the information that the patients glean from the Web may or may not be accurate.

The first half of this book contains definitions and explanations regarding the Internet as well as a history of the Internet. Read further and discover the best way to connect to the Internet, how to find information that you want on the World Wide Web, and explanations of common surgical uses of this new technology. The perils of using the Internet, including viruses and computer crashes, are covered. Discussions of continuing medical education and clinical trials online and the hot topic of telemedicine also are included. Finally, the use of electronic mail in a medical setting and the creation of a personal Web page for surgeons are described. The chapters are not written to logically follow each other, but instead to be independent sources of information. Use these as reference tools.

Along with several of my colleagues at the Royal Brisbane Hospital in Queensland, Australia, I did a study that examined the quality of information about laparoscopy on the World Wide Web. In reviewing these Web pages, we found several examples of dangerously false information about common surgical procedures. In many instances, these were merely typographical or transcriptional mistakes. We also found that many Web pages having a primary focus of laparoscopy contained no patient directed information. Of the pages that attempted to be educational, we determined that 70% contained statements that were controversial or misleading. In addition to "honest mistakes," there are some products, available only on-line, that are purely fraudulent. At present, there is limited regulation of what is displayed on medical Web pages. Web sites for products claiming to cure cancer through herbs or vitamins unfortunately are allowed to co-exist in cyberspace with Web pages for traditional organizations such as the American College of Surgeons (www.facs.com). For these reasons, I have compiled, for the second half of this book, a selection of Web pages that contain quality information directed at patients and/or surgeons. Here, you will find an annotated listing of reputable Web pages divided by specialty. In many instances, these would be good sites to refer patients when they want reasonable information about specific illnesses, procedures, or organizations. Nonmedical Web sites worth visiting are also included.

I truly hope you find this book useful. When writing it, I tried to identify certain areas in my day-to-day life that I think have been improved by the Internet. Enjoy!

Jeff W. Allen, MD
Department of Surgery
University of Louisville
Louisville, Kentucky

Contents

Foreword   **v**

Series Preface   **vii**

Preface   **xi**

1. What Is the Internet? 1
   The World Wide Web 1
   Web Pages 2
   Browsers 3
   Electronic Mail 4
   File Transfer Protocol (FTP) 4

2. History of the Internet 5
   Shot Heard 'Round the World 5
   Packet Switching 5
   ARPA Becomes DARPA 6
   Protocols 7
   World Wide Web 9
   Current Access 9
   Looking to the Future 9

3. What Can the Internet Do for Me? 10
   Initial Resistance 10
   User-Friendly Context 10
   What Can the Internet Do for Me? 11
      Electronic Mail 11
      Chat Rooms 12
      Telemedicine 12
      E-commerce 13
      Patient Information 13
      Personal Home Page 13

4. Connecting to the Internet 14
   What You Need: Computer, Modem, Monitor, Telephone,
   Internet Service Provider 14
      A Tale of Two Computers 14

Desktop Versus Laptop 15
The Parts of the Machine 16
The Need for Speed 16
Advanced Surfing 18

5. All That Glitters Is Not Gold 20
Misguided Patient Information Web Pages 20
"Caveat Viewor" 21
Computer Glitches 22
Viruses 23
Chat Rooms 24
Pornography 24

6. Finding the Information You Want 26
Viewing a Web Page 26
Needle in a Haystack 27
Search Engines 27
Alta Vista 27
Google 28
Hot Bot 29
Yahoo! 29
Search Tips 30
Order 31
Getting Cataloged 31

7. Clinical Trials, Literature Searches,
and Telemedicine 33
Clinical Trials 33
Available Online Studies 34
Literature Searches 35
Advanced Surfing 36
Telemedicine 37
Teleconsulting 38
Telesurgery 38
Telementoring 39

8. Electronic Mail 41
What You Need 41
Attachments 43
SPAM 43
Medical Applications of E-Mail 44
Guidelines for Medical E-Mails 45

The Worst- and Best-Case Scenarios When Guidelines for
Medical E-Mails Are Followed and Are Not Followed
     by Surgeons 46
  Advanced Surfing 50

9. Chatting Online 52
  Chat Rooms 52
  E-mail Lists 53
  ICQ 53
  Yahoo! Messenger 54
  NetMeeting 55
  Internet Telephony 55

10. Continuing Medical Education 58
  Online Advantages 58
  Start Earning Credit Hours 59
     Medscape 59
     HELIX 61
     CME Web 61
     Medconnect 62
     Pain 62
     University of Washington CME 62
  Conclusion 62

11. Becoming a Presence on the Web 63
  Everybody's Doing It 63
  What to Include 63
  Production 64
  Servers and Getting the Information to Them 65
  Homemade Web Pages 66
  Web Pages by Template 67
  Conclusion 68

12. Web Page Resources by Surgical Specialty 70
  Bariatric Surgery 70
  Cardiac and Thoracic Surgery 72
  Colorectal Surgery 75
  General Surgery 77
  Genitourinary Surgery 81
  Hand Surgery 84
  Minimal Access Surgery 86
  Neurosurgery 88

Orthopedic Surgery 91
Otolaryngologic Surgery 93
Pediatric Surgery 96
Plastic and Reconstructive Surgery 97
Transplant Surgery 99
Trauma Surgery 102
Vascular Surgery 105
General Surgery Products 107

13. Health-Related Internet Resources 111
General Medicine 111

14. Nonmedical Web Pages 114
Sports 114
News 115
Music 115
Cinema 115
Travel 116
Maps and Directions 117
Stock Market and Investing 117
All-In-One 118

Appendix I. Web Pages for Departments of Surgery in the United States   **119**

Appendix II. International Domain Suffixes and Common Top-Level Domains   **125**

Glossary   **130**

Index   **137**

1
What Is the Internet?

The World Wide Web
Web Pages
Browsers
Electronic Mail
File Transfer Protocol (FTP)

No other technology has influenced modern civilization as rapidly as the Internet. In only 5 years, the number of people connecting to the Internet has increased from 1 million in 1992 to over 16 million in 1997 worldwide[1]; A November 2000 study by NUA (www.nua.ie) Internet surveys estimates 167 million users in Canada and the United States alone.[2] In many areas of the world today, people with access to the Internet outnumber those who do not have access. The Internet affects each of us in some way each day. For surgeons to fully utilize the potential of the Internet, it is important first to address the simple question, What is the Internet?

The Internet is a large, interconnected network of computer users. It has evolved into an international system of computer networks in which users at any single computer on any particular network can conceivably exchange data with any other computer on any other connected network. There is no discrete physical location of the Internet; instead, it resides on a fluctuating portion of existing public telecommunication networks, predominantly telephone lines.

There are also many distinct components that make up what is collectively known as the Internet. These include the World Wide Web (WWW), Web Pages, browsers, electronic mail (e-mail), and the File Transfer Protocol (FTP). In reality, all of these are applications of the Internet.

The World Wide Web

The WWW is the portion of the Internet using the Hypertext Transfer Protocol (HTTP). This protocol allows diverse computers, operating languages, and systems to view Web pages in a common, flexible way. The essence of HTTP is that files can contain references to other files, and their selection will elicit a request to transfer information. This is the linking process that can be seen on nearly every Web page. The WWW is the area of the Internet that allows text and graphics to be displayed simultaneously by one computer program. That program is known as a Web browser, or browser for short.

Web Pages

A Web page is the collection of text, graphics, sound, and multimedia files that are displayed, on demand, by a browser. The Web pages are written in Hypertext Markup Language (HTML). The address where a Web page resides is known as the Uniform Resource Locator (URL). This information can be manually inputted into a browser so that one may visit a particular Web page. URLs have a constant, specific format. For example, the Web page for the popular search engine Yahoo! (Figure 1.1) is located at

http://www.yahoo.com

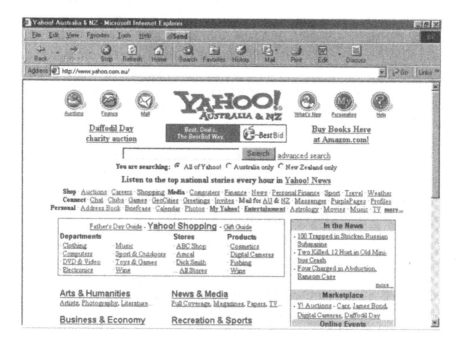

FIGURE 1.1 Yahoo! Australia displayed on Microsoft Internet Explorer.

URLs have five main components:

http://	Hypertext Transfer Protocol.
www	World Wide Web or other networks.
yahoo	The unique, main part of the URL; often a company name.
com	Commercial. One of the suffixes that follows the main portion of the URL. These also are known as "top-level domains."
————	Country suffix. When none present, United States (US) is default.

Yahoo! is now operational in Australia. The URL for Yahoo! Australia is

http://www.yahoo.com.au

Note that "au" is the two-letter country suffix for Australia. (For a list of country and top-level domains, see Appendix II.)

The top-level domains indicate the general content of the Web page as well as imply ownership. The most common, ".com," represents a privately or commercially run Web page. Others include ".gov" (government) and ".edu" (educational). Apart from .com and .net (network infrastructure) domains, there are restrictions to content associated with many of these categories.

A Web site is synonymous with a Web page; technically, however, a Web page may be viewed offline, whereas Web site denotes an online connection. "Home page" also may be used synonymously with Web page, although it usually refers to the first in a series of linked documents within a Web page.

Browsers

The software programs that allow Web pages to be fetched, displayed, and interacted with are called browsers. Examples of browsers include Microsoft Internet Explorer and Netscape Navigator. Many of the newer browsers will display a desired Web page when abbreviated URLs are typed in. For example, typing in "sunbeltmelanoma.com" will cue the Web page to display **http://www.sunbeltmelanoma.com** (Figure 1.2). Some browsers, such as Netscape Navigator version 6.0, will display the page when only "sunbeltmelanoma" is typed in.

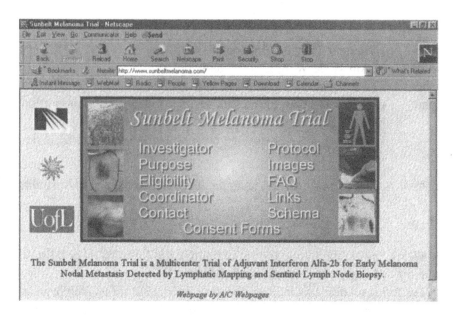

FIGURE 1.2. The Web page for Sunbelt Melanoma Clinical Trial, located by typing in "sunbeltmelanoma." (Reprinted with permission from Dr. Kelly McMasters, Sunbelt Melanoma Trial.)

Electronic Mail

The heaviest usage of the Internet comes from electronic mail. E-mail is the exchange of computer-generated messages by telecommunication. Messages sent via this technology are delivered more rapidly and, often, more reliably than those sent by regular mail. E-mail is generally delivered to the recipient within seconds of transfer by the sender. Accordingly, the old-fashioned letter, envelope, and stamp method now is known as "snail mail." E-mail is covered in detail in chapter 8.

File Transfer Protocol (FTP)

This is one of the simplest ways that individual files are exchanged between two or more remote users using the Internet. One of the most frequent uses of FTP is the transfer of Web page files from their creators to a computer that acts as their host or server. Another common use of FTP is downloading entire programs onto a computer for later use.

References

1. http://www.pbs.org./internet/timeline/.
2. http://www.nua.ie/surveys/how_many_online.

2
History of the Internet

Shot Heard 'Round the World
Packet Switching
ARPA Becomes DARPA
Protocols
World Wide Web
Current Access
Looking to the Future

The birth of the Internet was not a single event. Instead, the network now known as the Internet was shaped by a series of technological advances made by government, business, science, and academia. The modern Internet represents limitless benefits from a continuing commitment to research by public government and private industry.

Shot Heard 'Round the World

The catalyst for the creation of the Internet occurred on October 4th, 1957, when the Russian-built Sputnik became the first artificial satellite to successfully orbit the earth. Americans reacted intensely to this monumental feat performed by "the enemy" during the Cold War. Former President Harry Truman felt that the persecution of American scientists during the McCarthy era allowed the Soviets to pull ahead in the development of satellites and rockets. In response to Sputnik, the American government created the National Aeronautics Space Administration (NASA) and Advanced Research Project Agencies (ARPA).

Packet Switching

ARPA consisted of researchers who could investigate and develop technologies that were too risky to be left to entrepreneurs in the private sector. One of the technologies embraced by ARPA scientists was called "packet switching." This concept was developed by Leonard Kleinrock in 1961 at the Massachusetts Institute of Technology (MIT). Packet switching de-emphasizes hub systems and allows information to travel multiple routes. It has been likened to a fishnet, where each string of the net is a possible direction of movement (Figure 2.1). Packet switching was particularly important to the Department of Defense during the Cold War because there was a prevailing fear of a devastating nuclear strike by the Soviet Union. The theory was that a decentralized system of disseminating information would continue to function even if one or more key military locations had been destroyed by a Soviet warhead.

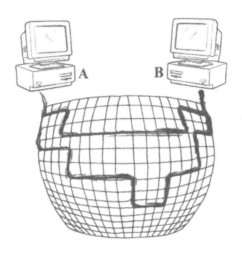

FIGURE 2.1. Packet switching allows multiple routes of travel from computer A to computer B, similar to traveling along the strands of a fishnet.

Packet switching was quickly applied to information travel in the civilian realm. The vision of a "galactic network" of globally interconnected computers using this technology belonged to J.C.R. Licklider of MIT, the head of the computer research program at ARPA. In 1969, ARPAnet was created by the ARPA scientists in an attempt to make Licklider's dream of a global network a reality. ARPAnet connected various academic and military sites that utilized the redundant packet switching system. Developments with ARPAnet also included a protocol that allowed dissimilar computers to communicate in a generic way.

ARPA Becomes DARPA

In 1972, ARPA had evolved into and was renamed the Defense Advanced Research Projects Agency (DARPA), and the Network Control Protocol was created to transfer data between hosts running on the same network.

Later, another protocol, called the Transmission Control Protocol/Internet Protocol (TCP/IP), which allowed diverse computer networks to interconnect with each other, was developed by DARPA scientists. Although it took over a decade to put TCP/IP into common use, its power and versatility continue to be of use today. This interconnected network represented the primitive Internet. The next decade was characterized by individual and often unrelated growth of local area networks (LANS), personal computers (PCs), and workstations.

Protocols

On January 1, 1983, the ARPAnet protocol was changed over to TCP/IP. At this time, the network was being used by a significant number of research, development, and operational organizations within the Department of Defense. Programmers at the University of Wisconsin created the Domain Name System later in 1983. This was an application for the packet switching technology that allowed the packets of information to be directed to a domain name instead of a numeric address; thus, the foundation for today's World Wide Web was laid. That same year, Microsoft unveiled Windows, which allowed users of the software to view and interact with multiple application programs simultaneously.

As personal computers became progressively more user friendly and affordable, the number of people with access to the new network grew.

On October 24, 1995, the United States Federal Networking Council unanimously passed a resolution defining the term *Internet* as follows:

Internet refers to the global information system that
  (i) is logically linked together by a globally unique address space based on the Internet Protocol (IP) or its subsequent extensions/follow-ons;
  (ii) is able to support communications using the TCP/IP suite or its subsequent extensions/follow-ons, and/or other IP-compatible protocols; and
  (iii) provides, users, or makes accessible, either publicly or privately, high level services layered on the communications and related infrastructure described herein."[1]

The increased availability and ease of connection to the Internet, coupled with the continuing decline in the price of personal computers, led to a dramatic increase in the use of the Internet in the 1990s (Figures 2.2 and 2.3). In 1991, the National Science Foundation lifted the restriction on commercial utilization of the Internet, which opened a new frontier in commerce, advertising, and product propagation. The number of people with access to the Internet has grown from thousands in the mid-1980s to millions in the late 1990s to hundreds of millions in 2000.

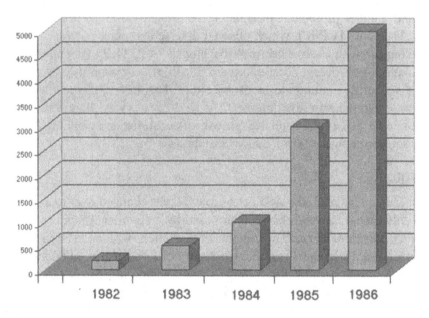

FIGURE 2.2. Growth of Internet users worldwide from 1982 through 1986. (Source for data: **http://www.pbs.org/internet/timeline/.**)

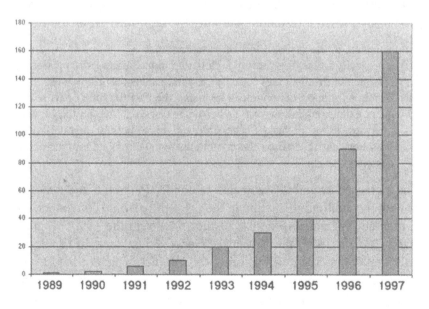

FIGURE 2.3. Growth of Internet users worldwide from 1989 through 1997 in hundreds of thousands. (Source for data: **http://www.pbs.org/internet/timeline/.**)

World Wide Web

In 1993, the phrase "World Wide Web" was coined in Switzerland. The World Wide Web, or WWW, represents the portion of the Internet allowing text and graphics to be shown simultaneously in a user-friendly format. Programs, called browsers, are created to fetch and display the documents containing text and graphics, which are now known as World Wide Web pages (Web pages for short).

Current Access

At present, the number of people who potentially have access to the Internet is difficult to measure, but it is clearly in the hundreds of millions. Many public libraries offer an Internet hub, as do nearly all universities. Soon, the number of people in developed nations who have the ability to use the Internet will outnumber those who do not. In 1998, it was estimated that 79 million Americans had access to the Internet.[2] Increasing numbers of patients obtain supplemental health-care knowledge through information obtained from Web pages. The number of people in America who use the Internet to seek medical information has climbed from 7.8 million in 1996 to over 30 million in 1999.[3]

Looking to the Future

The future of the World Wide Web undoubtedly will consist of smaller computers, more rapid data transfer, and greater mobility and flexibility of computer use. Soon, many, if not all, financial transactions will occur digitally. A digital medical record eventually will follow suit. The practice of medicine, specifically surgery, is sure to be affected by the ever-changing Internet. A glimpse into the current use of the Internet in surgery is described in the chapters that follow.

Referencess

1. **http://www.fnc.gov/internet_res.html**.
2. **http://www.infotechtrends.com**
3. Internet Medicine 1999;7:1.

3
What Can the Internet Do for Me?

Initial Resistance
User-Friendly Context
What Can the Internet Do for Me?
    Electronic Mail
    Chat Rooms
    Telemedicine
    E-commerce
    Patient Information
    Personal Home Page

Initial Resistance

Throughout history, fads in technology have come and gone with little impact. Remember flash-in-the-pan technologies such as eight-track tape machines, Betamax video systems, and laser disc players? With this in mind, many people were reluctant to quickly and wholeheartedly embrace the Internet. First-generation personal computers were difficult to use and nearly impossible to update, had a high price tag, and came with little or no working software. A modem was an expensive piece of optional equipment that transferred data between computers at a snail's pace. The initial resistance to the "Information Superhighway," as the Internet was originally known, is therefore not unfounded.

User-Friendly Context

Second- and third-generation computers are easier to use and much more affordable than their predecessors. Instead of seeing a "C-prompt" when the computer is turned on, users now get "point and click" Windows or MacIntosh screens that highlight operating systems that are easy to learn and use. Computers now come equipped with modems that readily connect to the World Wide Web, an extremely user-friendly part of the Internet. With the ease of connection and current ubiquity of the Internet, we can answer the question, "What can the Internet do for me?"

What Can the Internet Do for Me?

The answer is, everything and nothing. As pointed out by Smith[1] in *The Internet for Physicians*, the World Wide Web is so large and all-encompassing that information vital to the commerce of large corporations commingles with fraternity humor, and each can be retrieved and examined with similar ease. Popular uses of the World Wide Web today include getting stock quotes and trading, getting weather updates, and television listings, reading news and sports stories, buying and selling merchandise, and making travel arrangements. Specific to the field of medicine, literature searches, clinical trials, patient resources, and continuing medical education are frequent applications. None of the uses listed above is unique to the Internet. Each also may be done in the "old-fashioned" way.

What the Web does is to markedly simplify access to each of these areas and countless other applications by making them available from a personal computer. The convenience of doing a literature search, making reservations for the least expensive and most convenient airline travel, and arranging a hotel room at 10:00 P.M. from your home exemplifies the power of the Internet. While each of these could be accomplished without the use of the Internet, it could not be done in the few minutes it takes to do them on-line. Also, these tasks would likely require a trip to the medical library (if it is even open at 10:00 P.M.) and phone calls to multiple airlines and hotels (with the expected "on hold" telephone delays).

In addition to centralizing and simplifying, the Internet also offers some features that are unique. These include electronic mail, chat rooms, Internet telephony, real-time video conferencing, the rapidly expanding field of telemedicine e-commerce, patient information sites, and personal home pages.

Electronic Mail

Electronic mail (e-mail) has changed the way that people communicate. E-mail is quicker, easier, cheaper, and more versatile than mail sent with an envelope and stamp. Files containing graphics, sound, or video may be attached to the e-mail. This includes the ability to attach portions of a medical record to the e-mail, a likely future application.

Chat Rooms

Chat rooms allow many users to communicate with each other simultaneously in large on-line forums, usually segregated by topic. For instance, there is a chat room for patients with renal cell carcinoma located at **http://www.kidneycancerassociation.org**. Typically, the chats take the form of typed-text dialogue between users. Internet telephony is beginning to take this technology even further. By using sound cards, microphones, and speakers, the dialogue can take the form of the spoken word. Adding a video camera enables real-time video conferencing.

Telemedicine

The field of telemedicine is not entirely new or unique to the Internet. In fact, many hospitals routinely utilize some form of telemedicine in their day-to-day operations, most commonly in the diagnostic radiology department. Teleradiology allows digital images of radiographs to be stored and forwarded to a physician for interpretation remote from where the images were obtained. Usually, this requires special software on both the sending and receiving ends as well as a dedicated connection apart from a standard Internet Service Provider. The Internet will soon begin to bear the burden of telemedicine transmissions and is currently limited only by quality of graphics, bandwidth, and unfamiliarity of use by physicians.

As more physicians have become comfortable using the Internet, more services have become available. At some hospitals, physicians are able to view their patients' laboratory, radiology, and pathology reports by visiting the hospital's Web page.

Telemedicine is sure to become a dynamic part of the practice of medicine in this new century. Using an Internet connection and a high-resolution video camera, the entire world can have access to specialists no matter where they are located. Fields such as dermatology and cardiology, where diagnoses may be audio or video dependent, are good examples. While surgery has been performed on a patient by a surgeon at a remote site, this is unlikely to be the source of the most benefit from telesurgery.

Instead, telementoring, in which senior surgeons watch a video screen of an ongoing operation and guide less experienced surgeons located a distance away, has tremendous utility. The fields of laparoscopy, arthroscopy, thoracoscopy, and endoscopy are well suited to telementoring. This is made possible by sending the on-line video image from these procedures over the Internet so that the "telementor" may make suggestions or even assist in the operation using instruments on his or her desk attached to a robotic arm on the remote end.

E-commerce

Once filled with the buzzwords *untapped resources, unlimited growth potential,* and *unique investment opportunity,* E-commerce has now settled into its role in the American economy. E-commerce is simply the use of the Internet to conduct business. Many banks and credit cards offer their services on-line. The amount of merchandise available for purchase on the Web is staggering. Large e-tailers sell books (for example, Amazon at **http://www.amazon.com**), prescription medicines (Drug Store.com at **http://www.drugstore.com**), music (CD Now at **http://www.cdnow.com**), and much more.

Patient Information

A number of reputable organizations provide patient-directed Web pages with useful information. The American Heart Association (**http://www.americanheart.org**), the Crohn's and Colitis Foundation of America (**http://www.ccfa.org**), and Support for People with Oral and Head and Neck Cancer (**http://www.spohnc.org**) are good examples. On these Web sites, patients may find answers to questions about their diagnoses and review the personal stories of others who have already experienced treatment. Good Web pages exist for nearly every disease.

Personal Home Page

As described in Chapter 11, there are benefits in having a Web page for your practice. In addition to on-line advertising of services, a physician's personal page can help better inform patients. Office hours, timing of prescription refills, and "what to watch for" sections often are valuable. There also is an element of "keeping up with the Joneses." Nearly one-third of American doctors have their own Web page to detail their practice.

Reference

1. Smith RP. The Internet for Physicians, 3rd ed. New York: Springer-Verlag, 2002.

4
Connecting to the Internet

What You Need: Computer, Modem, Monitor, Telephone,
Internet Service Provider
    A Tale of Two Computers
    Desktop vs Laptop
    The Parts of the Machine
    The Need for Speed
Advanced Surfing

What You Need: Computer, Modem, Monitor, Telephone, Internet Service Provider

A Tale of Two Computers

To get online, a few pieces of electronic equipment, known as hardware, are necessary. A personal computer (PC) is first and foremost. PCs come in many shapes, sizes, brands, and price ranges. Two brands are commonly used: the Apple and the International Business Machines (IBM) computers. Technically, although Apple and IBM are brand names, they also represent a genre of computer. Most PCs fall into either the IBM or Apple genre. Compaq, Hewlett Packard, Packard Bell, Dell, Gateway, NEC, SONY, and many others are members of the IBM genre, and are often referred to as "IBM clones." These computers use similar operating systems and software (programs) and, for the most part, are interchangeable. While very few Apple "clones" exist, software that functions on Apple computers generally is incompatible with the IBM genre. The IBM computer and its clones generally use the Windows operating systems, manufactured by Microsoft.

Like a spirited college football rivalry, the line that separates Apple and IBM enthusiasts may divide friendships, households, and even marriages. Be that as it may, either type of computer, equipped with a modem and with the help of an Internet Service Provider (ISP), will allow its user access to the World Wide Web.

14

Desktop Versus Laptop

Personal computers are either laptop or desktop. Laptops are small, portable computers that generally trade convenience, mobility, and all-in-one design for limited features (Figure 4.1). Desktop computers are component-based machines that are larger, more powerful, and easier to add-on to or modify (Figure 4.2). Either may allow the user to access the Internet.

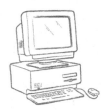

FIGURE 4.1. A laptop computer.   FIGURE 4.2. A desktop computer.

After deciding what genre of computer is right for you (Apple or IBM), the issue of mobility should be addressed. Laptop computers (also referred to as notebooks) allow on-the-go computing. Using a rechargeable battery, a laptop may be used anywhere, e.g., on an airplane, in an airport, and in hotel rooms. In fact, many slide shows at local and national scientific meetings emanate from laptop computers connected to a special projector.

A cellular phone and a modem combined with a laptop computer will permit Internet access from nearly anywhere in the world. Furthermore, airline manufacturers are beginning to place high-speed satellite connections to the Internet on newly built jet airliners, further facilitating online access during air travel. As laptop computers progressively become smaller and faster, portable, pocket-sized global Internet access machines will be developed.

However, there are a number of drawbacks to and limitations with laptop computers. First, they are considerably more expensive than their desktop counterparts. You will pay up to 50% to 100% more for a laptop than a similarly equipped desktop computer. Second, laptops are much less flexible with respect to upgrading or adding a component. Finally, the viewing screen, which is connected and flips up, is usually inferior to standard desktop monitors in image quality.

The choice between a laptop and a desktop is best made by considering the expected use of the computer. If you need a machine to access the Internet, send and receive e-mail, view daily stock quotes, and occasionally conduct a medical literature search, you would probably be better off with a desktop computer. However, if you need one for word processing while on the go, reviewing and updating reports for business meetings, displaying slide show presentations, or just passing the time on a transcontinental airline trip, you probably will be best served by a laptop. Don't fret too long on this decision. Many people eventually get both desktop and laptop machines for their computing needs.

The Parts of the Machine

Regardless of type, brand, or genre, a PC typically includes a hard drive, compact disc–read only memory (CD-ROM) or digital video disc (DVD) drive, floppy disk drive, keyboard, microprocessor, mouse, and a monitor.

The hard drive is the area where information is stored permanently or long-term; it is "invisible" to the user. In contrast, a floppy drive allows data to be written on a removable disk that fits in one of the computer's bays. Most experts recommend that important data be stored on both the hard drive and a floppy disk. A printed copy (known as a hard copy) is a good idea as well. A keyboard allows typed information to be entered. The mouse controls the position of the cursor on the screen. The microprocessor executes the commands of the computer and runs the software. Random access memory (RAM) temporarily stores important information for rapid retrieval.

Optional accessories include a sound card that enables music, voices, and sounds to be generated and "played" by the PC; a video or graphics card that displays high-resolution on-screen images; and a printer that creates paper copies (hard copies). A monitor, although usually sold separately from a PC, is a mandatory piece of equipment that displays everything on a viewing screen.

The modem, short for "modulator-demodulator," allows computers to share information with each other by way of a standard telephone line. Most preassembled computers sold today have a built-in modem. The modem will connect, via a telephone line, to an Internet Service Provider (ISP). The ISP is a company that provides its customers access to the Internet (usually for a monthly fee). Many universities offer a free or discounted provider for student and faculty use. To summarize: a PC equipped with a modem, a telephone line, and an ISP are needed to connect to the Internet.

The Need for Speed

A speedy connection to the Internet may seem like a luxury, but it is really important to many computer users. Waiting three or four minutes for a simple Web page to load onto the screen is unacceptable for most people, especially busy professionals such as surgeons.

Three factors limit the speed at which a Web page, or any online file, may be viewed: (1) the speed of the modem, (2) the capacity of the computer, and (3) the connection rate of the ISP. The latter is perhaps the most important. How fast the ISP delivers the data to your computer is variable. On computers that run Windows, this information is easily found by moving the mouse's cursor over the connection icon at the right lower corner of the screen (Figure 4.3).

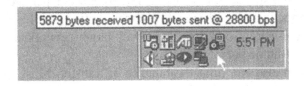

FIGURE 4.3. The cursor is shown just to the right of the connection icon.

Currently, most ISPs operate at 56 kilobits per second (Kbps); 56 Kbps means that, in each second, 56,000 bits are sent to the computer. (Table 4.1 explains bits and bytes.) If a large online image is about 63,000 bytes in size, it would take approximately 9 seconds to download it at 56 Kbps from the Internet onto a computer.

TABLE 4.1. The size and speed of things.

Unit	Definition	Example
Bit	The smallest unit of computerized data	A single digit number in base 2 (0 or 1)
Byte	A set of bits (usually 8) that make up a character	The letter A
Kilobit	1,000 bits	Modems commonly move information at 56 kilobits per second (Kbps)
Megabyte (MB)	Approximately 1 million bytes	A standard floppy disk contains about 1.4 MB of memory space
Gigabytes (GB)	Approximately 1,000 Megabytes	A computer's hard drive often contains about 10 gigabytes of memory space

Many ISPs operate at 56 Kbps until they reach maximum capacity of number of clients online; then they automatically will log on users at a slower speed, often 28.8 Kbps. Integrated Services Digital Network (ISDN) connections, which are becoming more common, operate faster, and cable modems are faster yet. An ISDN connection will transfer data at a rate of around 128,000 bits per second, or 128 Kbps.

Quicker transfer of information will occur with a T1 connection, at over 1,540,000 bits per second. The T1 and cable modem connections usually require special hardware, and this speed of data transfer is not possible with standard modems and phone lines. These T1 connections are usually part of a much larger network, such as a university, and are usually not for individual home use. T3 lines, the next generation of superfast connections, transfer data at a rate of 44,736,000 bits per second, quick enough to effectively broadcast a full-screen motion picture on the Internet. Again, these are usually part of a much larger network and not practical for the at-home user.

The modem also can limit the rapidity of transfer. Most modems today operate at 56 Kbps, the maximum speed of the standard ISP. This means that the modem handles data as fast as the ISP delivers it. An older modem, with a maximum speed of 33.3 Kbps or 28.8 Kbps, will not handle the higher data transfer speed of a quicker ISP. This will slow transmission and cause Web pages and graphics to load much more slowly.

Finally, the computer's microprocessor and RAM can significantly affect the speed of transmission. Text and images from frequently visited Web pages will be stored in RAM so that they do not need to be reloaded with each new site visit. The more RAM available, the more that can be stored and the less that has to be loaded from scratch with each visit. The processor of the computer regulates the overall speed of computations by the PC. A quicker processor will move through a series of Web pages at a much higher speed than a computer with a slower processor. It also will respond to commands more quickly, with less of a lag.

In summary, then, to get online it is necessary to have a personal computer equipped with a modem, a telephone line, and an Internet Service Provider. A variety of options are available with each component. The fastest Web-surfing experience will come with a top-of-the-line computer equipped with a fast processor, more than ample amounts of random access memory, a dedicated telephone line, and an Internet Service Provider with a large capacity of users or a cable connection. However, a slower, less expensive machine with a standard provider certainly will get the job done.

Advanced Surfing

Even smaller than the laptop computer is the hand-held computer, also known as the personal digital assistant (PDA). These devices are typically small enough to fit into a pocket and have many of the same features as their larger counterparts. Some have a tiny keyboard that allows information to be entered, but most accept handwriting as input using a wand, an input window, and the Graffiti writing system. PDAs commonly are used for maintaining schedules and contacts, and for doing simple calculations.

Most PDAs can interface with larger "base" machines, such as a desktop personal computer. In this way, a synchronization occurs, and information from both devices is shared. Notes taken from a medical conference onto the PDA, for example, are put into the desktop machine at a specified location. Similarly, appointments entered into the desktop machine now appear in the PDA's datebook. In addition, many PDAs now allow wireless Internet access, so sending and receiving e-mail and accessing Web pages is possible.

There are a number of helpful medical programs that can be placed onto a PDA and are available for free download from many Web pages. One is the drug reference guide from ePocrates (**http://www.epocrates. com**). By following the step-by-step instructions, the guide can be downloaded onto a desktop or laptop computer and then synchronized with the PDA. The guide is easy to use and contains an alphabetical list of medications. Categories describing adult and pediatric dosing, contraindications, drug interactions, adverse reactions, and cost, and individually entered notes are available for each medication.

A similar drug reference is available from Medscape (**http://www.medscape.com**). The Medscape Web pages also contains other tools for a physician's PDA under the heading "Medscape Mobile." They include an article reader and medical calculator. The calculator contains formulas for over 50 clinical values, such as body mass indicator, Ranson's criteria, alveolar-arterial oxygen gradient, anion gap, and cardiac output. By entering the variables, the program will calculate the desired value and even store it in a database for future reference. The article reader works by first downloading a group of articles ("Medscape Surgery Journal Scan") and then transferring them to the PDA at the next synchronization. Each journal scan contains numerous abstracts from large peer-reviewed surgical journals. Since the PDA can be taken almost anywhere, the abstracts go with it and can be read at any free moment (between cases in the doctor's lounge, etc.).

5
All that Glitters Is Not Gold

Misguided Patient Information Web Pages
    "Caveat Viewor"
Computer Glitches
Viruses
Chat Rooms
Pornography

Millions of people visit millions of Web pages each day and are treated to an amazing array of on line features and functions. Perhaps the most powerful feature is sheer information propagation. There is no better way to "get the word out" than by using the World Wide Web or by delivering it using e-mail. Health care is certainly no exception—it, too, is an industry that wants to get its message out. In fact, medicine is probably one of the most frequently visited topics on the Internet, with one in three Americans in 1999 using the Internet to obtain medical information.[1] At present, however, there is no means of assuring that what is presented on health-related Internet sites is scientifically valid. In addition to a large number of misleading Web pages, the Internet is host to a number of evil entities, such as viruses, hackers, and computer crashes. Villains, con artists, and stalkers find a home on the Web as well. All that glitters on the World Wide Web is not gold, and some suggestions for protecting yourself are presented in this chapter.

Misguided Patient Information Web Pages

As presented at the 2000 meeting of the Society of American Gastrointestinal Endoscopic Surgeons, Web pages with a focus on laparoscopy were found to contain recommendations that were considered false or misleading 70% of the time.[2] Errors were merely typographical or transcriptional in some instances, but in other instances the controversial opinions of the Web page authors were presented as fact (Table 5.1).

TABLE 5.1.
Types and examples of errors found on Web pages about laparoscopy.

Type of error	Example
Typographical	The gallbladder stores bile which you do not need.
Transcriptional	During laparoscopic cholecystectomy, the common bile duct is clipped and ligated.
Opinion presented as fact	The Veress needle is an uncontrolled harpooning device.
Overzealous promotion of laparoscopy	There really is no pain associated with laparoscopic cholecystectomy.

"Caveat Viewor"

Even worse than typographical or transcriptional errors about a scientifically proven operation is the online advertisement of unproven treatments for serious medical illnesses, especially cancer. The Federal Trade Commission (FTC) has investigated many Web sites offering cures for diseases that simply do not work. Legal settlements with several of these companies have been reached. However, the number of Web pages advertising nontraditional medical services is staggering, and it is unrealistic to expect the FTC to effectively police them all.

As pointed out by Dr. James Anderson in *MD Computing*, some Web pages are difficult to shut down because they sell legal products, such as Laetrile, a compound made from apricot seeds. Claims that the seeds are "the answer to cancer" are not true, but the ambiguous wording makes prosecution difficult. Such false claims of miracle cures prompted Dr. Anderson to coin the phrase *"caveat viewor"* (let the viewer beware) when dealing with online medical Web pages.[3]

In general, most patients who look online will find good, well-meant medical information. However, except for a handful of online journals, none of the information is peer-reviewed. One of the best ways to guide your patients to quality Web pages is to personally read and review some of the sites that concentrate on your area of surgery. Record the sites that you believe contain helpful information and offer them to patients who ask for this information. Better yet, put them on your personal Web page in a "Selected Links" section.

Computer Glitches

Imagine this scenario: You are working late in your office polishing off your presentation for a conference tomorrow. You have meticulously added intraoperative photographs taken with your digital camera. You have written text that surely will qualify for a special category of the Pulitzer Prize. You have filmed, edited, and digitized video footage of a new technique you have invented that may revolutionize the way surgery is performed in the future. Just before you are about to save this multimedia masterpiece, you see an all-too-familiar blue screen with the message, "Your computer has experienced a 0D fatal exception at module 09932109 and will shut down."

In all likelihood, this is the end of the line for this computing session. All unsaved work is absolutely doomed, including your presentation. Even though personal computers have become advanced, efficient, and reliable computing machines, they occasionally "lock up" for no apparent reason. It seems that the more bells and whistles there are on your computer, the more likely it is to lock up. Often, strenuous computing tasks, such as "burning" a disc (creating a music CD), printing a large file, or capturing a video stream, can catalyze a freeze. This is especially true when these activities are taking place at the same time or when multiple other applications are "open."

There really is no avoiding or explaining these painful experiences. Occasionally, your computer will give warning signs of an upcoming lock-up and allow you quickly to save your work and restart the computer. Most glitches, however, occur without warning. While there is no way to avoid these freezes, the damage that they inflict can be minimized by saving your work at 10- to 15-minute intervals.

Even worse than the temporary computer freeze is the all-out crash. This may at first look like the simple lock-up, but, as you try to restart your computer, there are signs that things are desperately wrong. The normal computer screen will not come up or the cursor does not respond to moving the mouse. The result is that no matter what you try, your computer will not operate normally. This is "digital armageddon."

The most common causes of computer crashes are viruses and power surges. The good news is that both of these major contributors to computer crashes are preventable. A good surge protector can eliminate power surges. (My monitor was struck once by lightning, but the surge protector saved my computer and the data on its hard drive.) Antiviral software is helpful in eliminating viruses, but safe downloading techniques (described below) are perhaps more important.

Like the lock-up, sometimes there is no avoiding a computer crash. Unlike the lock-up, however, a crash usually erases your hard drive and potentially a lifetime of work. The strategy to combat this is to back up your work frequently on floppy disks or CD-ROMs. Unfortunately, viruses can spread from your computer to a disk or CD-ROM. Printed copies of important documents, therefore, should be made to help immunize yourself from the hazards of an all-out crash.

Viruses

Like their biologic counterparts, computer viruses are small, pathogenic entities with a great capacity to spread and infect. Unlike the natural strain, however, computer viruses are man-made with the sole purpose to cause harm. Technically, they are disguised programming code that causes some unexpected, unpleasant event. The damage that a virus can inflict is variable, ranging from an unknowing small occupancy of memory to a nuisance scrolling message to a complete computer meltdown. Some viruses are immediate in their effect, whereas others are dormant until a specific time, date, or other cue awakens them.

Viruses are transmitted in a number of ways. Frequently, they come attached to e-mails, but almost always require activation by the person receiving it. For this reason, you should *never open an attachment to an e-mail from someone you do not know.*

Even if you know the sender, care should be taken because some viruses work by invading the e-mailing program and, unbeknownst to its host, sending out e-mails to everyone in the address book. So, your friend Harry may send you an e-mail with an attachment and a generic subject line like "check this out!" You open it, and now you, too, are infected. You may not even know it immediately. If you question Harry, he will say he never sent the e-mail or knew he was infected. By this time, though, many of the contacts in your e-mail address book will have received an e-mail from you with an attachment and the generic message "check this out!" It is in this way that viruses rapidly can be spread.

Similarly, downloading files or programs from the Internet can be hazardous. At present, it is not possible to "catch" a virus by merely visiting a Web site. There must be some willful download of a product or file. Finally, floppy disks and CD-ROM may be infected and serve as formites for transmission.

The best defense against a computer virus is to know the origination of every file and program that you place into your computer. Since this is not always practical, most people rely on antiviral software to detect viruses and prevent them from infecting their computer. Demonstrations of antiviral software may be seen and downloaded from McAfee (**http://www.mcafee.com**) and Symantec (**http://www.symantec.com**).

Chat Rooms

There have been reported examples of people feigning physical illness in disease-dedicated chat rooms.[4] These mentally ill people exhibit a form of online Munchausen's syndrome. They experience some personal emotional gain, reveling in the fact that others believe that they have a serious disease. Unfortunately, the imposters use information gathered online about the disease to make their stories more believable.

Another group of untruthful people are those who have misrepresented other aspects about themselves in chat rooms and attempt to arrange a physical meeting with their chatting buddies. Often, this begins innocently enough with the exchange of a telephone number or address. However, this situation can rapidly deteriorate and, in general, is to be avoided. This is not to say that every chat room is filled with villains and stalkers; however, except in special circumstances, it is best to restrict communications, especially those that are medically related, to an anonymous form.

Pornography

It is probably unrealistic to attempt to keep teenagers from visiting one of the most popular areas of the Internet, those with an explicit sexual theme. Just as the Internet offers convenience and centralization of many useful features for the productive citizen, it also makes it easier for adolescents to download pornography. There are software systems, including Cyber Sitter (**http://www.cybersitter.com**), that recognize sexual content in Web pages, newsgroups, and e-mail and prohibit access to selected users. Other similar products are Cyberpatrol (**http://www.cyberpatrol.com**), Surf Watch (**http://www1.surfwatch.com**), and the Internet Content Rating Association (**http://www.icra.org**).

The way that these programs function is to detect key words within Web pages and prohibit visitation of pages containing these words. Unfortunately, some of the words that trigger the block are included in medical Web pages that should not be blocked. These include "breast" in breast cancer, "sexually" in sexually transmitted diseases, and so forth. Many of the programs have a password-protected override feature that allows adults to access any page, including those that are blocked based on word content.

References

1. Louis Harris Poll, 1999. Americans Seek Health Information Online. Also **http://www.louisharris.com**.
2. Allen JW, Finch RJ, Nathason LK, O'Rourke NA, Fielding GA. The poor quality of information about laparoscopy on the World-Wide-Web. Oral and poster presentations, SAGES, Atlanta, Georgia. March 29, 2000.
3. Anderson JG. Health information on the Internet: let the viewer beware (Caveat Viewor). MD Computing 2000; July/August:1921.
4. Stephenson J. Patient pretenders weave tangled "Web" of deceit. JAMA 1998;280:1297.

6
Finding the Information You Want

Viewing a Web Page
Needle in a Haystack
Search Engines
    Alta Vista
    Google
    Hot Bot
    Yahoo!
Search Tips
Order
Getting Cataloged

Viewing a Web Page

The conventional way of viewing a Web page begins by typing its address into the browser and then hitting the "Enter" button. This Web page address is known as a Uniform Resource Locator (URL). This simple way to find what you want depends on knowing the URL of the Web page in the first place. We are bombarded daily by Web page addresses in magazines, on television commercials, billboards, and other forms of advertising. Often, these URLs are seemingly obvious. It is easy to predict that to visit the Web site for the Pepsi Cola company, one would type in **http://www.pepsi.com** (Figure 6.1). However, many of the Web pages have complex names such as the hypothetical **http://www.mycompany.com/sales/newlistings**. Not only are these addresses impossible to remember, but they are troublesome to write down and often not inherently obvious by the content of their name.

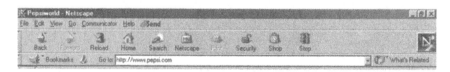

FIGURE 6.1. Typing in a known URL.

Needle in a Haystack

There are countless millions of pages available on the Web today, and this number is rapidly increasing. These pages cover nearly every subject under the sun—from surgery to geography to horse racing. Given the large number and variety of topics of the Web pages, it is not surprising that finding information on any specific subject can be quite difficult. A hunt for a Web page about laparoscopic repair of a recurrent inguinal hernia, for example, may be like finding a needle in a haystack in a field of haystacks.

Search Engines

Search engines eliminate these time-consuming, blind quests for Web pages about specific topics. Search engines are specialized Web pages that attempt to "index" the World Wide Web. If the conventional way of typing in a known Web page address is not possible, search engines can help. They will list all sites in their database that match certain key words or phrases. A visitor to a search engine can type in words describing the desired subject material, and the search engine will display all matching Web pages.

Different search engines perform these matches a bit differently. Some specialize in finding images, sound files, or video clips. Some work well with broad topics, while others effectively weed out larger topics and match only narrow terms. A few search engines are described below.

All search engines are helpful, and there are many more available than are reviewed here. Many offer a personalized home page, with the respective search engines having a centralized role. Examples include My Yahoo, My Lycos, and My Alta Vista. On these personalized pages, not only are the search functions available, but stock portfolios, travel itineraries, calendars, and breaking news stories are also available.

Alta Vista

Alta Vista, which means "the view from above," was founded in 1995, and today it is a subsidiary of the Compaq Computer Corporation. Alta Vista is an exceptionally fast and comprehensive search engine. It is available in 25 languages and contains eight unique search functions. A search for a topic such as "laparoscopic inguinal hernia repair" will return all Web pages in the Alta Vista database containing all four of the key words first, then Web pages containing three of the four words, and so on. The preferences section of Alta Vista allows activation of features that describe the listed Web pages. These include the date the page was last modified, size of the page, and what language the page uses.

Google

One of the newer search engines that is becoming quite popular is Google (**http://www.google.com**). Google offers no-nonsense searching from a large and powerful database (Figure 6.2). There is limited extraneous material at this Web site, and the engine is very fast. What makes Google even nicer is the language, display, and filtering options. By clicking on one of these, the user can make alterations to the search functions. A language constraint may be selected, which will then cause the engine to return only Web pages written in a desired language. The number of results listed per page may be changed and this affects the speed of the search engine, with fewer results per page making for a faster search. The optional "safe search" feature of Google will block Web pages that contain pornographic content from appearing in search results.

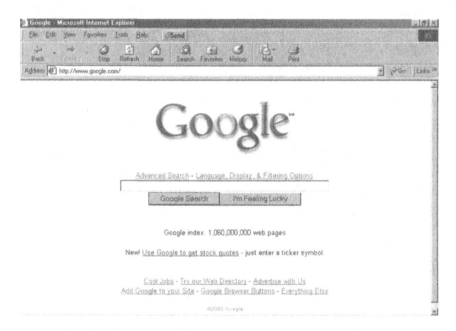

FIGURE 6.2. The simple look of Google. (Reprinted with permission from Cindy McCaffrey.)

Google is different from other search engines that rely on keywords or meta-search technology to catalog the Web. Google uses a patent-pending technology called PageRank that tries to select the most important, relevant pages first. Google also offers some unique, advanced features like "who links to you." This allows a Web page to be typed in, and Google will determine which sites in its database link to that page. For Web masters, it is a helpful and powerful tool.

HotBot

Although not as prominent as some of the other search engines, HotBot (**http://www.hotbot.com**) is powerful and extremely user-friendly. Hot-Bot won awards from *SmartMoney*, *PC Magazine*, *PC Computing*, *PC World*, *New Media*, and CNET for the best search site. It has sophisticated search features and an easy-to-use interface. HotBot prides itself on indexing every word, active link, and media file on the more than 110 million Web documents in its database. In addition, it refreshes and updates this entire database at least once a month.

Yahoo!

Possibly the most recognized brand name on the Internet, Yahoo! was the first online navigational Web page. It was founded in 1994 by David Filo and Jerry Yang, who were Standford University Ph.D. students at the time. Filo and Yang created a Web page to keep track of their personal interests on the Internet. Today, Yahoo! is a global Internet commerce and media company with a market capitalization of $59.4 billion.

The Yahoo! search engine is category based (Figure 6.3). For instance, a recent query using the keyword "surgery" returned 281 category matches. Categories included plastic surgery, gynecologic surgery, etc. More than 2,390 Web sites were listed with a total of 406,000 matches for individual pages.

However, in the Yahoo! system, desired pages often are not found within the categories, and thus its usefulness as a search engine is decreased. For instance, when the search phrase "laparoscopic surgery" was entered, only one category matched, and it was for "Health > Medicine > Surgery > Hysterectomy." There were, however, 51 individual Web sites that matched but were considered outside this category.

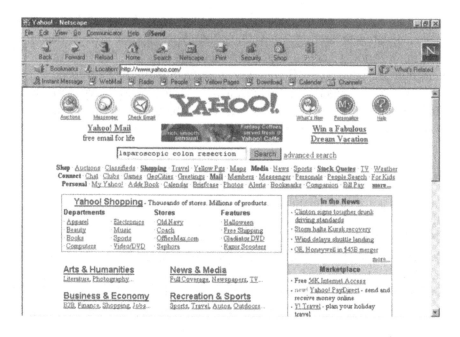

FIGURE 6.3. Yahoo! at work.

Search Tips

While search engines are designed to make Web experiences more pleasant by eliminating time spent looking for unknown Web pages, they, too, can be time-consuming. Here are a few tips to help you with your searching experience:

1. Do not stray from the path. While searching for "laparoscopic splenectomy," do not click on links about the really slick, new laparoscopic tools available for use in an inguinal hernia repair. Stick with one topic, and visit the other one during a later session.
2. Use very specific search phrases first. If there are no matches, then broaden your key words. For instance, do not look for a specific type of proton pump inhibitor by searching for "GERD." A Google search for "GERD" found over 379,000 matches. Instead, search for "medical management of GERD" (21,000 matches) or "proton pump" (17,900 matches).
3. Use capital letters for proper names and punctuation makes liberally. Using quotation marks around a phrase often will alert the engine that you want only Web pages with that entire phrase. Searching for Michael Jordan will target any Web page with Michael or Jordan, while

searching for "Michael Jordan" will require both names to be present and in that order. Anything that you can do to decrease the number of unwanted matches is to be encouraged.

4. Search engines can be used to find Web pages as well as sounds and graphics.

5. Use language and date restrictions when these are available options. A page about a certain surgical technique is useless if written in a language you are unable to read.

6. Some engines recognize + and − signs. "Beef + stew" requires that both words appear in listed Web pages, while "beef − stew" will return all pages that contain "beef" except those containing both "beef" and "stew."

Order

Given the large number of Web pages a search engine will provide on a specific topic, the order in which they are listed becomes progressively more important. If the query "Denver Cosmetic Surgery" has 8,000 Web pages that match, it is virtually useless to be number 7,999 on the list. It would be unlikely for a consumer to sift through 7,998 pages in order to get to that one.

The pecking order for now matching Web pages are listed is different for each search engine. Various engines handle this delicate situation differently. Lists may be ordered by seniority, by highest percentage of matched words, or by frequency of visits. Some engines will list certain Web pages high on their list based on reciprocal links to the search engine, advertising sponsorship of the search engine by the Web page, and other dubious criteria.

Getting Cataloged

Finding Web pages of interest on a specific subject is made easier with a search engine. However, how does the search engine know where all those Web pages are? This is a pertinent bit of information because it influences how *you* can get *your* Web page indexed. (For more information on building a Web page for yourself or your practice, see chapter 11.)

There are two ways that engines catalog the World Wide Web. The first is the easiest. Most search engines have a special area that allows owners or administrators of a Web site to submit their page for consideration of inclusion into the engine's database. There usually is an "add

URL" button, and clicking on this button is how a request to include this Web page in the search engine is initiated.

The second way that a Web page is included in a search engine's database is through "spiders." Spiders are drone-like computer programs that seek out and record Web pages, their location, and their content. The sole purpose of a spider is to methodically visit these Web pages, record their key words and subject matter, and report these results back to the search engines. In this way, unbeknownst to its administrators, a Web site may be added to the database of a search engine.

Given the number of search engines currently available (hundreds or even thousands), it is a laborious process to register your Web page with all of them. It also can take a prohibitively long time to be "spidered." This has led a few companies to fill this niche by offering registration services to numerous search engines for a small fee. An example of this may be seen at **http://www.submitit.com**.

7
Clinical Trials, Literature Searches, and Telemedicine

Clinical Trials
    Available Online Studies
Literature Searches
    Advanced Surfing
Telemedicine
    Teleconsulting
    Telesurgery
    Telementoring

Clinical Trials

Therapeutic decision making in nearly every field of medicine is based on evidence obtained in previous clinical trials. These trials frequently are fraught with labor-intensive paperwork and discarded data due to nonadherence to study protocols. The traditional way of accruing these data includes filling out and mailing or faxing the study forms, a word-of-mouth spread of information about the trial, and limited immediate study feedback to participating patients and physicians about the progress and results of the study.

Some centers conducting trials have been able to network their data and share it with other institutions. This has increased patient accrual, decreased the work involved in obtaining data, and provided a resource of information for trial patients and investigators. A global network, such as the Internet, has the capacity to markedly change the scope of clinical trials in all fields of medicine. Specifically, use of the Internet can facilitate randomization, patient and physician recruitment, data entry, and distribution of trial progress and results.

International multicenter trials are now feasible using the Internet. Electronic correspondence eliminates significant lag times associated with overseas mail. A much larger patient population with widespread demographic variation is available with an international online study.

Available Online Studies

The Clinical Trials Resource Center (**http://pharminfo.com/conference/clintrial/ct_rsc.html**) is available online and includes an international listing of more than 5,200 clinical trials that are actively recruiting patients. Basic information about trials is directed toward patients, and frequently asked questions are addressed.

The National Institutes of Health (NIH) has a "Search the Studies" Web page located at **http://clinicalstudies.info.nih.gov**. At this time, a viewer can type in a diagnosis, sign, symptom, or other keyword, and the NIH database will return all current clinical trials that match. Each trial lists its title, a summary, its sponsoring institute, recruitment details, exclusion and eligibility criteria, and contact information.

Two other similar resources are Center Watch (Figure 7.1) (**http://www.CenterWatch.com/main.htm**) and Clinical Trials.gov (**http://www.clinicaltrials.gov**).

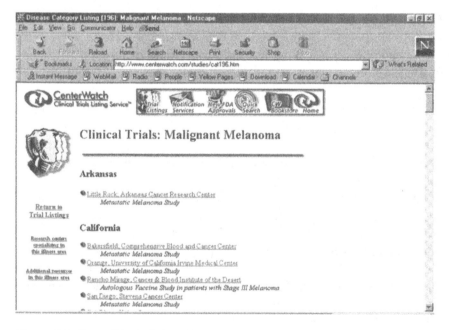

FIGURE 7.1. Center Watch listing of melanoma trials. (Reprinted with permission from Dan McDonald, Center Watch.)

In addition, some of the larger, well-funded clinical trials have a dedicated Web page. An example of this is the Sunbelt Melanoma Trial (**http://www.sunbeltmelanoma.com**) (Figure 7.2).

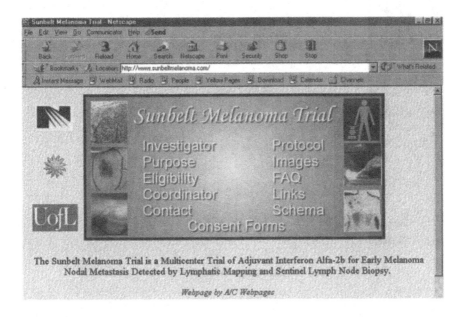

The Sunbelt Melanoma Trial is a Multicenter Trial of Adjuvant Interferon Alfa-2b for Early Melanoma Nodal Metastasis Detected by Lymphatic Mapping and Sentinel Lymph Node Biopsy.

Webpage by A/C Webpages

FIGURE 7.2. The Web page for the Sunbelt Melanoma Trial. (Reprinted with permission from Kelly McMasters, MD, Sunbelt Melanoma Trial.)

Literature Searches

One of the first medical applications of the Internet was the online literature search. Today, the World Wide Web offers effortless searches of the medical literature. Numerous educational organizations and private corporations fund Web pages that offer free searches of the Medline database. At present, these include PubMed (**http://www.ncbi.nlm.nih.gov/PubMed**), MedPortal (**http://www.medportal.com**), Healthgate (**http://www.healthgate.com/medline/search-medline.shtml**), and Medscape (**http://www.medscape.com**) to name just a few. On these Web pages, the abstracts for articles written in the past 20 years are available. In many cases, entire articles can be ordered and purchased. This is especially helpful for manuscripts in hard-to-find journals and in cases where interlibrary loan is slow. PubMed is shown in Figure 7.3.

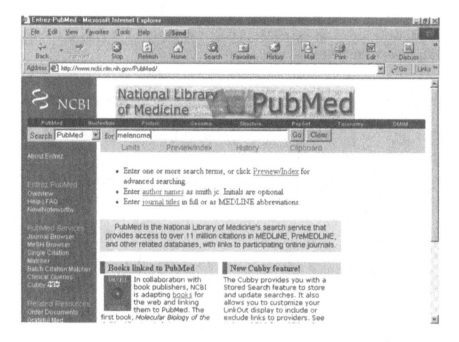

FIGURE 7.3. Pub Med beginning a Medicine search of melanoma.

Of the Web pages listed above, perhaps the best is Medscape. Membership permits unlimited and reliable Medline searches and a personal Web page. The Medscape literature search offers highly customized options from 1960 to the present and includes journal articles.

Advanced Surfing

The World Wide Web rapidly is becoming the preferred media for the literature search. Prior to the age of the Internet, searches of the medical literature required a trip to the closest health science library, performance of the search (often by paging through a series of books), finding the journals, and photocopying the articles. This was especially cumbersome for those practicing in a rural area, as libraries in small hospitals are limited in the number of journals they carry. Now, abstracts, and in many instances full-length articles, are available from any computer terminal connected to the Internet.

However, experience using the Web pages that search the Medline database is needed, or this, too, becomes a daunting task. The creation of a proper "search phrase" is paramount for success. The search phrase is what you type into describe the subject that you are researching. Many of the Web pages that offer a search of the Medline database listed above use "Natural Language Searching" (NLS). With this system, the Web page will find all articles that contain any of the words in your search phrase.

For instance, the search phrase "chronic angina" will cause the Web page to list all articles containing the word "chronic" and all the articles listing the word "angina." Obviously, this list will contain the few articles that contain both "chronic" and "angina." Because the Web page is set up to know that you probably want the articles containing both "chronic" and "angina," these are generally listed first. To eliminate the articles having one but not the other phrase, simply change the search phrase to "chronic and angina." However, this search still will include an article that has the word "chronic" in its title and "angina" in the text of the abstract.

This has demonstrated how to focus your literature search more narrowly. In some instances, you will want to broaden your search. For instance, when searching on the subject of laparoscopic colectomy, many articles will be missed if the search phrase is simply "laparoscopic and colectomy." This is because authors use different words to describe the same procedure. For instance, an article titled "Colon Resections Through the Laparoscope" would be missed using the search phrase "laparoscopic and colectomy." One way to avoid this is to use truncated words and an asterisk in your search phrase. Try "laparo* and col*." The search will return all those articles that contain words beginning with laparo and those beginning with col. In this way, laparoscopic, laparoscopy, and laparoscope are combined with colon resection, colectomy, and colorectal to give you a large set of articles from which to choose.

Telemedicine

The ability to "store and forward" clinically related text and images has made the field of telemedicine possible. Telemedicine is the delivery of health care and the sharing of medical knowledge using telecommunication systems.[1] At present, only a small fraction of telemedicine is performed over conventional telephone lines via the Internet, while most is based on dedicated networks.

Telemedicine has unlimited applications. For example, it has been used to deliver health care to underprivileged areas of the world. In remote areas where needed specialists are often unavailable, hospitals have used telemedicine systems in dermatology, cardiology, pathology, endoscopy, and radiology.[2] Interactive control of glucose control and fetal monitoring have been reported.

Teleradiology has been available for over 20 years and is in place in many hospitals nationwide. Currently, it is the most common form of telemedicine in use. In fact, many tertiary centers now have "filmless" radiology departments, instead relying upon onscreen radiographic images. Many satellite emergency departments depend on a connection to a larger center with a radiologist employing telemedicine techniques. In theory, this will help make radiologic diagnoses faster and lead to quicker initiation of treatment.

Telemedicine is helpful in assisting in the selection of patients for triage to tertiary care centers. In the traumatic neurosurgery realm, this system has been shown to be safe and cost-effective by Bailes et al[3] and others. In some instances, transportation to and from a hospital is the most costly aspect of patient care. The use of telemedicine can similarly determine which patients may be treated at a distance and which should be transferred to a larger, specialized facility. This has been applied in the medical care of prisoners.

Finally, patient follow-up, especially in areas where transport to the nearest physician is difficult, is feasible online. DeBakey and colleagues[4] have used the Internet to follow a patient who underwent mitral valve replacement in the United States and returned to Russia after the operation. The patient's medications, electrocardiographs, and activity status were reviewed in the U.S. via the Internet, and specific clinical recommendations were made while the patient remained in Russia.

Teleconsulting

Using telemedicine for medical consultation is "teleconsulting." Teleconsultations will ensure that no area in the world equipped with an Internet connection will be without needed specialists. Norway was the first country to implement a fee schedule for teleconsultations, a scenario in which medical opinions are rendered by a consulting physician at a distance from the patient. Starting in 1999, United States physicians performing teleconsultations were compensated financially for their services. Initially, such consultations have been limited to patients who live in rural, underprivileged areas and require that the referring physician be physically present.[1] As patients and doctors become more comfortable with this setup, this field of medicine is sure to grow.

Telesurgery

Telesurgery involves the use of telecommunications to facilitate performance of an operation. Telesurgery is especially applicable in the fields of laparoscopy, endoscopy, and arthroscopy because all rely heavily on visual rather than tactile cues. During a conventional laparoscopic procedure, surgeons view a monitor and manipulate their hands on instruments traversing the abdominal cavity. Although some sense of touch is used, the surgeon relies more heavily on depth perception and visual stimuli.

On August 29, 1996, a laparoscopic procedure was broadcast "live" on the Internet.[5] Surgeons in the United States and Argentina actively discussed portions of the laparoscopic cholecystectomy while the case was ongoing. This Web broadcast brought up many questions about surgery online, namely: Is it ethical, useful, and safe to actually perform surgery over the Internet?

Already, however, the envelope is being pushed. Using robots and the Internet, laparoscopic procedures have been performed by surgeons at a distance from their patient.[6] By manipulating handles connected to a computer in command of instruments inside a patient's abdominal cavity, Dr. Franco Favretti performed a laparoscopic gastric band in 1999 from a distance of 6 feet from the patient; this is perhaps the first account of true telesurgery.[6]

There are a host of problems with using telesurgery to operate on a patient from a distance. The first is access. As technology improves, the distance between the patient and the surgeon will lengthen. Technicians with the patient will need to obtain intraabdominal access for the instruments. Often, this can be one of the major sources of morbidity in the procedure. Having a fully trained surgeon placing the access ports nullifies the benefit of a surgeon at a distance.

As the distance between patient and surgeon crosses state lines, a licensing issue surfaces. Should the surgeon be required to have a license in the state where the patient is located? A busy "telesurgeon" would need licenses in nearly every state. Furthermore, what licensing is required when the transmission crosses international borders?

The issues of complication management and conversion to open surgery also are important. Unless the technicians standing by the patient are able to handle potential catastrophes (like major vascular injuries), the setup is not safe. A conversion from laparoscopic to open-site surgery is needed when there is a concern that the case cannot be safely completed using minimal-access techniques. Again, this need for an experienced local surgeon nullifies much of the benefit of telesurgery.

Telementoring

Perhaps more practical than performing an entire operation at a distance is the concept of surgical telementoring. In this scenario, an experienced surgeon (mentor) guides less experienced surgeons through difficult portions of a procedure. This is done using oral and visual commands while watching the progress on a computer monitor.[7] The telementoring concept has been shown to be a safe, potentially cost-saving system for training surgeons in advanced laparoscopy.[8]

One of the most interesting examples of surgical telementoring took place aboard the U.S.S. Abraham Lincoln. While the ship floated in the Pacific Ocean, five laparoscopic inguinal hernia repairs were performed on naval seamen under shore-based telementor guidance.[9] Telementoring has been reported to be useful in other clinical scenarios including complex ophthalmologic, urologic, and neurologic procedures.[10–12]

References

1. Strode SW, Gustke S, Allen A. Technical and clinical progress in telemedicine. JAMA 1999;281(12):1066–1068.
2. Stephenson J. Physicians find teleactivity hot near the North Pole. JAMA 1998;280(15):1296.
3. Bailes JE, Poole CC, Hutchison W, Maroon JC, Fukushima T. Utilization and cost savings of a wide-area computer network for neurosurgical consultation. Telemed J 1997;3(2):135–139.
4. Aucar JA, Doarn CR, Sargsyan A, Samuelson DA, Odonnell MJ, DeBakey ME. Use of the Internet for long-term clinical follow-up. Telemed J 1998; 4(4):371–374.
5. Gandsas A, Altrudi R, Pleatman M, Silva Y. Live interactive broadcast of laparoscopic surgery via the Internet. Surg Endosc 1998;12(3):252–255.
6. Cadiere GB, Himpens J, Vertruyen M, Favretti F. The world's first obesity surgery performed by a surgeon at a distance. Obes Surg 1999;9(2):206–209.
7. Schulam PG, Docimo SG, Saleh W, Breitenbach C, Moore RG, Kavoussi L. Telesurgical mentoring. Initial clinical experience. Surg Endosc 1997;11(10): 1001–1005.
8. Rosser JC, Wood M, Payne JH, et al. Telementoring. A practical option in surgical training. Surg Endosc 1997;11(8):852–855.
9. Cubano M, Poulose BK, Talamini MA, et al. Long distance telementoring. A novel tool for laparoscopy aboard the USS Abraham Lincoln. Surg Endosc 1999;13(7):673–678.
10. Camara JG, Rodriguez RE. Real-time telementoring in ophthalmology. Telemed J 1998;4(4):375–377.
11. Lee BR, Caddedu JA, Janetschek G, et al. International surgical telementoring: our initial experience. Stud Health Technol Inform 1998;50:41–47.
12. Levine SR, Gorman M. "Telestroke": the application of telemedicine for stroke. Stroke 1999;30(2):464–469.

8
Electronic Mail

What You Need
Attachments
SPAM
Medical Applications of E-mail
    Guidelines for Medical E-mails
    The Worst- and Best-Case Scenarios When Guidelines for
        Medical E-mails Are Followed and Are Not Followed by
        Surgeons
Advanced Surfing

Electronic mail, also known as e-mail or email, has become an accepted and often preferred method of communication. Using e-mail, a person can easily correspond with one or many recipients. Often, transmission of data occurs in a matter of seconds or fractions of seconds. The majority of Internet Service Providers, such as America Online (AOL), include at least one (and often many) e-mail addresses with the purchase of their services. These e-mail addresses may be called POP3 accounts, mailboxes, identities, or a variety of other terms. Furthermore, free accounts may be obtained through companies such as Yahoo! (**http://www.yahoo.com**), Juno (**http://www.juno.com**), Hotmail (**http://www.hotmail.com**), or Medscape (**http://www.medscape.com**). These companies use their e-mail Web pages for advertising, and this pays for the cost associated with maintaining free e-mail accounts for others.

What You Need

Software, such as Microsoft Outlook Express, is required to send and receive e-mail (Figure 8.1). Many Web browsers (Microsoft Internet Explorer or Netscape Navigator, for example) may be configured to do this as well. Most of the free e-mail services (Yahoo!, Hotmail, etc.) may be entirely browser-based through a series of Web pages (Figure 8.2).

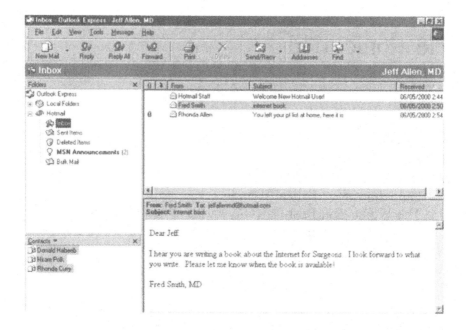

FIGURE 8.1. Outlook Express in action.

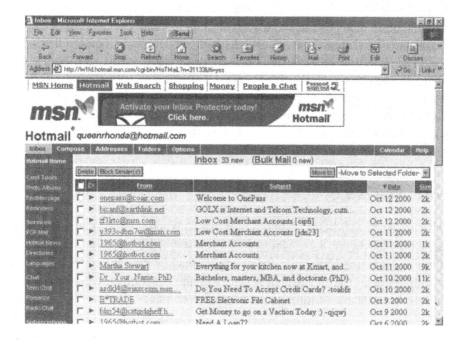

FIGURE 8.2. Hotmail requires only a browser to function.

Most IBM-type computers are equipped with Microsoft Outlook Express as part of their standard software. This simple but powerful program allows messages to be composed, sent, received, filed, deleted, or saved. Separate files may be attached to these e-mails. A "search" function allows individual words or phrases to be located within incoming, outgoing, or saved mail. An "address book" stores the names and e-mail addresses and is automatically updated with that information when a message is sent or received. This information also may be manually entered. One or a number of different e-mail accounts may exist within a single version of Outlook Express. Each account has a unique user with an individual password.

Another software program that may be used to manage e-mail accounts is Eudora (**http://www.eudora.com**). This company's shareware* product, Eudora Light, performs many features of Outlook Express and is available for download from the company's Web page. Eudora Pro is the high-end version and must be purchased as software or downloaded for a fee from the company's Web page.

Attachments

Both Eudora and Outlook Express allow files to be attached to outgoing or incoming e-mails, enabling the e-mail message to act as a sort of carrier pigeon. By selecting a file from your computer and clicking on the "attach" and "send" buttons, a file can be attached and sent. Attached files can be of almost any variety and are limited mainly by their size; larger "attachments" take longer to send or to be received. An attachment could be a graphic of a new sailboat, a spreadsheet with tax information for your accountant, or literally anything. In the future, we commonly will send attachments such as an electrocardiogram for a cardiologist to interpret or a high-definition image of a radiograph for the radiologist to examine at home. In many areas, this already is done on a daily basis.

SPAM

Currently, electronic mail constitutes the business area of the Internet. Unfortunately, much of this activity is known as "SPAM." In addition to being the celebrated, copyrighted meat product from Hormel, SPAM also

---

*Shareware is software distributed free of immediate charge on a trial basis.

refers to unsolicited e-mail. Essentially, SPAM is the e-mail equivalent of telemarketing. (The exact sequence of events that led unsolicited e-mail to become known as SPAM is not well defined, but may involve a famous Monty Python sketch about the product.)

Medical Applications of E-mail

Although much of the e-mail today is social in nature or SPAM, this exciting but simple technology has tremendous potential for physicians. Using e-mail, surgeons may communicate with patients and their families, colleagues, therapists, hospital administrators, visiting nurses, and insurers. It is not far-fetched to assume that nonurgent hospital ward calls and "beeps" will be replaced by electronic messages in the very near future. This likely will come to fruition when cordless Internet access to personal digital assistants becomes widespread. The Palm Pilot is an example of a personal digital assistant.

The current use of e-mail by surgeons has been curtailed by the fear that easier personal access will cause a bombardment of messages that will require a response.[1] Electronic mail has been shown to be a useful adjunct to postoperative follow-up after ambulatory surgery. Possible benefits include cost savings, ease in collecting quality improvement data, and the potential for increased reporting of unpleasant events, such as complications or patient dissatisfaction. Potential pitfalls of surgical e-mail follow-up include privacy and security concerns, and a possible delay in response to messages that may require emergent responses or actions.[2]

E-mail already has supplemented the traditional methods of doctor-patient communication in many surgical practices. It has the potential to enhance the professional relationship between physician and patient; however, in some instances, it also can worsen it. Patients may acquire their surgeon's e-mail address from a business card, letterhead, Web page, or by direct inquiry. If a physician has no intention of answering e-mail from a patient, his or her personal e-mail address should be removed from those venues. Not answering e-mail from patients is similar to not returning phone calls and should be avoided.

No matter how thoroughly an upcoming operation is discussed with a patient in the office, inevitably and expectedly additional questions will arise. E-mail offers a way for patients to ask these questions, and get a reasonable, well-thought out response. Since these e-mail inquiries do not require immediate responses, a surgeon can reply to them at a convenient time instead of the current practice of returning phone calls or beeps immediately when the nature of the situation is not known.

Guidelines for Medical E-mails

Certain guidelines should be employed when corresponding by e-mail with colleagues, patients, and families.[3] First, an e-mail address should be included in the patient's medical record.[4] Second, the exact identity of the recipient must be known prior to sending information that may be linked to the patient's private medical records. The e-mail address should be obtained in the office when the patient's telephone number, address, and other contact information numbers are obtained. This is to ensure that any communication goes solely to that e-mail address. The same discretion should be used when communicating by e-mail as when writing in the patient's chart.

There is a potential for misunderstanding the meaning of statements when using electronic mail instead of the spoken word. "Real time" communication nuances, such as word inflection and emotion, are not possible with e-mail. Clearly expressed thoughts should be used when communicating by e-mail. Questions posed as yes/no should be answered as such and liberally annotated with explanations.

Table 8.1 summarizes the ten recommended rules to follow when using e-mail with patients.

TABLE 8.1. Ten commandments for e-mail use with patients.

1. Set up one e-mail address designated solely for patient correspondence.
2. At the initial office visit, obtain the patient's e-mail address, if available.
3. Before answering e-mail from a patient, verify that the e-mail address matches the one obtained from the patient.
4. Answer e-mail personally and promptly when possible.
5. Remember the limitations of printed words. Emotion, inflection, and emphasis are eliminated. Use clear language that is concise and eliminates jargon.
6. E-mail should be treated as part of the medical record; lawyers, colleagues, and insurance companies ultimately may read it.
7. E-mail from a patient, especially in the immediate postoperative period, may indicate a problem. If this appears to be the case, make telephone or personal contact as soon as possible and document this.
8. Do not make diagnoses based on e-mails. Even if the patient has been recently treated in the office or discharged from the hospital, it is not possible to make a reliable diagnosis electronically.
9. Anxiously awaited test results, such as of a breast biopsy, are best handled by an office visit rather than by e-mail.
10. Retain a printed copy of all incoming and outgoing e-mail and place it in the patient's office chart.

The Worst- and Best-Case Scenarios When Guidelines for Medical E-mails Are Followed and Are Not Followed by Surgeons

Example 1

> To: Dr. Plastic Surgeon
> From: Aspiring Model
>
> Dear Dr. Plastic Surgeon:
>
> I am a little concerned about my incisions following my breast implant. Are there sutures that need to be removed?
>
> AM

> To: Aspiring Model
> From: Dr. Plastic Surgeon
>
> No, the stitches that I placed when performing your breast implant procedure were all subcuticular. They will dissolve in 2 to 3 weeks.
>
> Dr. PS

> To: Dr. PS
> From: Paparazzi Pete
>
> Aha, just as I suspected. Aspiring Model did have a breast enlargement procedure. The rumors are true, and I have it in writing from you. Do you have a glossy 8 × 10 of yourself that we can run with the story? I can't wait to see Aspiring Model's face when she realizes that her secret is out!
>
> PP

In this example, the surgeon did not verify the source of the e-mail message. The authentication process involves matching the e-mail address supplied by the patient and in the patient's files to the e-mail address to which the surgeon's e-mail is being sent.

Example 2

To: Dr. Cleverlap
From: Jill Stoneformer

Dr. Cleverlap

Thanks for taking the time to tell me all about my upcoming laparoscopic cholecystectomy. You mentioned that bleeding and infection are possible complications of this procedure. I forgot to tell you that I frequently take aspirin for chronic headaches. I take two or three a day. Should I stop them?

JS

To: Jill Stoneformer
From: Dr. Cleverlap

Mrs. Stoneformer.

I confirmed that your e-mail address matches the one you filled out on our office questionnaire. First, there are other possible complications with removing the gallbladder either through a laparoscope or in the open fashion. They include common bile duct injury, injury to the bowel by the instruments, risk of stroke or heart attack associated with the anesthesia, and the possibility of additional procedures or operations. Second, it would be a good idea to stop the aspirin for 2 weeks prior to the surgery to help minimize the risk of bleeding. Please e-mail me further if you have any questions. *Copy placed in patient's chart.*

In this example, the surgeon did everything right. He verified that it was, in fact, the patient who was requesting this information. The answer was clear, concise, and open-ended; more information is available if the patient has a need for it. A copy of the surgeon's e-mail was placed in the patient's chart.

Example 3

To: Dr. Clevelap
From: Nervous Nancy Norton

Dear Dr. C.:

Since you took my gallbladder out this morning I have had some pain around the incision, and it feels like I am having an attack of the colic that I had before the operation. What should I do?

NN

Dear Mrs. Norton:

It is not uncommon to have pain after laparoscopic cholecystectomy. Please take the pills I prescribed for you.

Dr. C.

To: Dr. Cleverlap
From: Nervous Nancy Norton

Dear Dr. C.:

I tried the pills that you gave to me, but they have made me sick to my stomach, and I vomited them up. Now my pain is worse since I can't keep them down, and I am nauseated. What should I do?

NN

To: Nervous Nancy Norton
From: Dr. Cleverlap

Dear Mrs. Norton

I will call in a prescription for your nausea and a different medicine for the pain relief.

Dr. C.

To: Dr. Cleverlap
From: Nervous Nancy Norton

The second medicine that you gave me has made me very drowsy. I can barely type at the computer. It hasn't touched my pain. This is the worst pain I have ever had in my life. I feel very faint. What should I do?

NN

To: Nervous Nancy Norton
From: Dr. Cleverlap

Dear Mrs. Norton:

I would stop taking the pills and see if you can sleep. If you can't, you may want to go to the emergency room and have them look you over.

Dr. C.

Note: Phone call to Dr. Cleverlap from Dr. Workatnight in the Emergency Room:

Dr. Cleverlap: I have your patient, Nancy Norton, in the emergency room. She is accompanied by her lawyer. She has a hemoglobin of 5.0 g/dL and appears in shock. She keeps mumbling something about three prescriptions for pain pills, and that you knew all about her worsening pain. Her lawyer is smiling and has copies of what appear to be some recent e-mails.

In this example, the surgeon did not realize early on that the patient's problems needed to be addressed in person. This problem should not even have been handled over the phone, let alone by e-mail with its inherent possible delays. Urgent or emergent problems should not be handled by e-mail.

Example 4

To: Dr. WW Savvy
From: Mr. Poor Protoplasm

Dear Dr. Savvy:

After you did my hernia repair through the scope, my scrotum has blown up like a balloon and my groin aches. The pain is really intense. Is this normal?

PP

To: Mr. Poor Protoplasm
From: Dr. WW Savvy

Dear Mr. Protoplasm:

It is normal to have pain after this operation, but it is impossible for me to examine you via e-mail. If the pain is worsening and is not being relieved by the pain pills I have prescribed for you, please call me and I will make arrangements to see you. An enlarged scrotum is a known side effect of laparoscopic hernia repair, and is usually due to air. However, if the scrotum is discolored and appears to be worsening or is causing pain not relieved by your pain medication, please call me and I will arrange to see and examine you.

Dr. S.

Copy placed in patient's chart.

In this example, the surgeon gives clear answers and offers the patient the opportunity to be seen. A copy of the surgeon's e-mail message is placed in the patient's medical record.

Advanced Surfing

In 1996, Congress passed the Health Insurance Portability and Accountability Act (HIPPA). This was designed to improve the process of health care reporting while establishing guidelines for electronic transfer of health information. Although in many ways HIPPA was originally written with an emphasis on claims and encounters transactions, it is applicable to electronic transfer of any portion of the patient medical record, including e-mail. HIPPA requires that all health plans and providers maintain safeguards to ensure confidentiality, integrity, and authenticity when they transfer patient data electronically.

With respect to e-mail, the best way to comply with HIPPA regulations is to encrypt all messages containing any patient data. Encryption is the conversion of data (text, graphics, etc.) into a form that cannot easily be understood without authorization. To send someone encrypted mail, you must have the recipient's digital identification (ID). Decryption, the conversion of the encrypted data back to its original form, also relies on a digital ID, and this is the authorization process. S/MIME (Secure Multi-Process Internet Mail Extensions) is an acceptable method of sending encrypted e-mail, and this system is included in the latest versions of the Web browses from Microsoft and Netscape and in the popular e-mail software Eudora and Outlook Express.

References

1. Brailer DJ, Hackett TS. Points [and clicks] on quality. Hosp Health Networks 1997;71(22):32.
2. Ellis JE, Klock PA, Mingay DJ, Roizen MF. Use of electronic mail for postoperative follow-up after ambulatory surgery. J Clin Anesth 1999;11(2):136–139.
3. Kane B, Sands DZ. Guidelines for the clinical use of electronic mail with patients. The AMIA Internet Working Group, Task Force on Guidelines for the Use of Clinic-Patient Electronic Mail. J Am Med Inform Assoc 1998;5(1):104–111.
4. Spielberg AR. On call and online. JAMA 1998;280(15):1353–1359.

9
Chatting Online

Chat Rooms
E-mail Lists
ICQ
Yahoo! Messenger
NetMeeting
Internet Telephony

Using existing phone lines and the interconnectivity of the Internet, it is possible to hold online conversations with others using the typed or spoken word. Chat rooms were perhaps the first to use this form of online communication. Recently, several companies have introduced products that facilitate these online conversations. One of the first was ICQ. Yahoo! Messenger and Microsoft NetMeeting followed. Most recently, Internet telephony was created, which allows online telephone conversations in a computer-to-telephone format. To fully utilize Internet telephony, your computer must be equipped with a sound card, speakers, and a microphone, in addition to the standard necessary equipment, including a modem.

Chat Rooms

Chat rooms are specialized Web pages where simultaneous communication between two or more people is possible. To access one of these chat rooms, simply type in its address in the browser. Chat room communication usually takes the form of typing messages back and forth or, in some cases, actually speaking into a microphone and hearing others through the computer's speakers. A number of people may be in a chat room at any one time, and they all can see everything that is typed. Chat rooms are public affairs and are not great places to hold one-on-one conversations. In fact, there are often multiple conversations going on simultaneously.

Chat rooms are often segregated by theme. The medical application of the chat room is in the form of online support groups, which are especially useful in uncommon diseases. Through discussion of diagnoses and treatment plans, practical tips on coping and emotional support become available.[1] At the Cancer Information and Support international Web page (**http://www.cancer-info.com**), there are chat rooms available for a variety of cancers. Examples of specific chat rooms include those for Ewing's sarcoma (**http://www.cancer-info.com/chat/ewings.htm**), multiple myeloma (**http://www.webspawner.com/users/myelomaexchange**), and glioblastoma (**http://www.cancer-info.com/chat/glioblastoma.htm**). In fact, there are chat rooms on the Internet available for most major diseases.

Chat rooms are not immune from the hazards of Internet usage. People feigning illnesses have been reported to reside in chat rooms. Exhibiting a form of Munchausen syndrome, these people appear to thrive on the attention and support afforded to them in these online support groups.[1] The abundance of disease-specific information available on the World Wide Web unfortunately gives people with factitious disorders medical details to support their claim and make their story believable.

E-mail Lists

Similar to chat rooms, e-mail lists are becoming popular as avenues for health care professionals to share practice parameters and discuss interesting or problematic cases.[2,3] These function as discussion groups but not in "real time." Instead, messages written by members of the list are distributed to subscribers on a regular basis, via e-mail. The requirement of a working e-mail address may discourage impostors in this type of forum.

ICQ

ICQ ("I seek you") is a powerful online communication tool that permits users to chat, send messages, or send files. To use ICQ, simply download the free software, located at **http://www.icq.com**, and install it onto your computer. Then complete a "buddies" list of people in whom you have an interest. ICQ will let you know which of your chatting buddies are online at any time and enable you to contact them. If one of your friends logs on while you are online, you will be alerted. The modes of communication available with ICQ are chat, voice, message board, data conferencing, and file transfer.

Yahoo! Messenger

From the makers of the Yahoo! search engine, Messenger is a powerful but simple tool that allows users to communicate with other registered Yahoo! users. The Yahoo! Messenger service has two ways to converse. First, instant messages allow users quickly to exchange the typed word with online friends. Unlike e-mail, instant messages appear as soon as they are sent and come through the Messenger software. Second, a voice conference can occur between two or more people. To initiate a conversation, move the cursor over the person's name and click on "start a voice conference" (Figure 9.1).

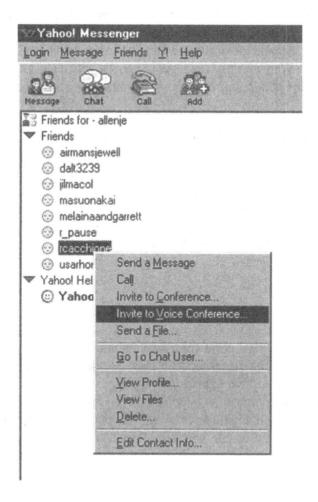

FIGURE 9.1. Initiating a voice conference.

Once an online chat has begun, simply click on the top button and speak into the microphone. Your voice is transmitted over the Internet to the people in your voice chat and is heard on their speakers. Your party or parties generally will hear you clearly. If one member of the group does not have a microphone, he or she may type a reply and everyone involved in the conversation will see it on their screen.

Messenger is free, reliable, and easy to use. In addition, special features include price alerts for your stocks, news, weather, and sports scores. The disadvantage of Messenger is that two people cannot talk simultaneously, and thus it does not simulate real conversation. A times, the program will "freeze," especially with heavy use. Also, since it is not an actual telephone conversation, a prearranged meeting time is necessary to reliably communicate. The Yahoo! Messenger software may be downloaded without cost at **http://messenger.yahoo.com**.

NetMeeting

NetMeeting is software that is similar to Yahoo! Messenger but has the added feature of integrating a video signal into the communication process. A video camera connected to the computer is needed to send but not to receive the video signal. Like Messenger, NetMeeting is a free service and requires a preset meeting time. However, unlike Yahoo! Messenger, use of NetMeeting requires a specific meeting place. NetMeeting use requires one to log on to a special server. While servers are free, they are frequently crowded and may be difficult to access. In addition, a much wider bandwidth is needed to send and receive the signal. Finally, unlike ICQ or Yahoo! Messenger, which have friend or buddy lists, NetMeeting merely lists your name on the server. Unsolicited telephone calls, especially from "shady characters" with pornographic screen names, are an occasional nuisance. The IBM version of Messenger may be downloaded at **http://www.microsoft.com/windows/netmeeting/download**.

Internet Telephony

The examples above illustrate online chatting between two or more people who are connected to the Internet and at a computer. Internet telephony requires only one user to be online. There are a number of companies that provide free PC-to-phone calls within the United States. Some offer these calls to other places in the world as well. This means that calling the United States (or selected foreign countries) from a computer anywhere in the world is free of additional cost.

Dialpad is an example of a company offering this service, and perhaps it was one of the first online (Figure 9.2). At present, it boasts that it has over 10 million subscribers. Dialpad, unlike ICQ, Messenger, chat rooms, and NetMeeting, allows a person who is connected to the Internet to place a direct telephone call to another person's telephone number. The previous examples all entail computer-to-computer communications. Internet telephony is thus very similar to a standard phone conversation. The person who is online speaks into a microphone and listens to the responses over the computer's speakers. The person who is speaking into the phone may not even know that the conversation is taking place over the Internet. Most of the companies generate advertising revenue by inserting online advertisements during the call.

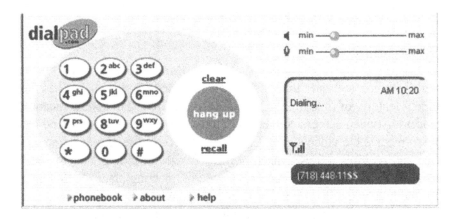

FIGURE 9.2. Dialpad places a call to New York from a user connected in Australia. (Reprinted with permission from Kevin S. Chou.)

Another example of a company that provides free Internet telephony is Go2Call (**http://www.go2call.com**). Recipients in the United States, the United Kingdom, Ireland, and Germany may be reached using this service. Go2Call also offers a Callfinder service. By typing in any telephone number worldwide, Go2Call will list Internet telephony companies that offer service to the area and what the call will cost on the respective services. Table 9.1 lists selected companies offering Internet telephony.

TABLE 9.1. Internet telephony companies.

Company	Web page	Free calling area
Dial Pad	**http://www.dialpad.com**	To U.S.
Go2Call	**http://www.go2call.com**	To U.S., Canada, U.K., Ireland, Germany
Media Ring	**http://www.mediaring.com**	To U.S., Canada, China
Net2Phone	**http://www.net2phone.com**	To U.S.
PC Call	**http://www.pccall.com**	None
Phone Free	**http://www.phonefree.com**	To U.S.

While Internet telephony is a wonderful and exciting advance in on-line communication, it has not completely revolutionized the way we make long distance telephone calls. There are a few reasons why. First, these Web pages often are overcrowded, and it can be difficult to place your call, especially at peak calling times. Second, the quality of the call is variable. In many instances, the call may sound as crisp and clear as a call on a standard telephone line. Often, however, it sounds more as if you were calling from a wind tunnel on Mars, with significant lag times, echoes, distortions, and gaps in transmission. Finally, it is best that the recipient expect the call. Often there is a one- to five-second delay at the very beginning of the call, and an unknowing recipient may hang up before the call can get started.

References

1. Stephenson J. Patient pretenders weave tangled "Web" of deceit. JAMA 1998;280(15):1297.
2. McLauchlan GJ, Cadogan M, Oliver CW. Assessment of an electronic mailing list for orthopaedic and trauma surgery. J R Coll Surg Edinb 1999;44(1): 36–39.
3. Gilas T, Schein M, Frykberg E. A surgical Internet discussion list (Surginet): a novel venue for international communication among surgeons. Arch Surg 1998;133(10):1126–1130.

10
Continuing Medical Education

Online Advantages
Start Earning Credit Hours
    Medscape
    HELIX
    CME Web
    Medconnect
    Pain
    University of Washington CME
Conclusion

Most health care professionals are required by their licensing board to stay current in their field. This is done to ensure that, after completion of formal training, they will continue educational activities and improve upon their knowledge, skills, and performance. In the United States, surgeons are required to obtain credit hours in what is known as continuing medical education (CME). Typical venues that count as CME credit include attendance at national society meetings, local lectures at accredited institutions, and self-study courses.

The number of CME credit hours awarded is roughly equal to the amount of time spent in the activity. The amount of mandatory CME varies by state. In Alabama, for example, 12 hours of credit are required each year. In Illinois, however, 50 hours of credit are mandatory each year. Some states spread the credit hour requirement over two or three years.

Online Advantages

The World Wide Web gives surgeons a new way to obtain required CME credits. This can be accomplished by visiting areas of CME Web pages known as modules. In general, each module includes lecture material fol-

lowed by a quiz. A passing grade on the quiz will earn its taker a specified amount of CME credits.

Online CME has advantages over the traditional way of accumulating
credit hours. First, it usually is much cheaper. Many CME Web sites have
modules that are free of charge. Others may carry a nominal price tag
($15 to $30). The cost of registration alone at national meetings is usually tenfold higher. In addition to the cost of tuition, travel expenses, and
lost wages, are associated with traditional CME. As well, it is impossible to put a price tag on the precious time spent away from home and
family.

The second advantage of online CME is its lack of time constraints.
National meetings and lectures are typically inflexible with respect to personal schedules. The Web, on the other hand, is open "24/7" and can be
accessed from the comforts of home. Often, a CME module does not even
need to be completed at one sitting.

The quality of an online teaching session frequently is superior to a
live lecture. This is because the online session usually is refined by cuts
and edits, similar to a motion picture. The finished product is much more
polished than a live lecture. The flexibility of HTML, the language of
Web pages, lets the CME modules take the form of slide shows or video
presentations as well as the form of standard on-screen text and graphics.

Start Earning Credit Hours

Medscape

The CME center at Medscape (**http://www.medscape.com**) is a good
place to start a quest for credit hours. Visitors must log in using their free
membership. There is a list of 21 categories containing CME modules.
General surgery, critical care, orthopedics, transplantation, and urology
are included.

In the module, the learning objectives and lecture material are presented
and then followed by a quiz covering the material. If a passing grade on
the quiz is obtained and a course evaluation completed, CME credit is
awarded (Figure 10.1). In many instances, an "instant certificate" is displayed. This may be printed out, thus, hard-copy proof of the CME is immediately available (Figure 10.2).

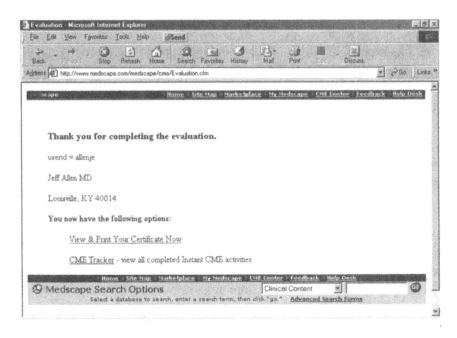

FIGURE 10.1. CME credit earned at Medscape.

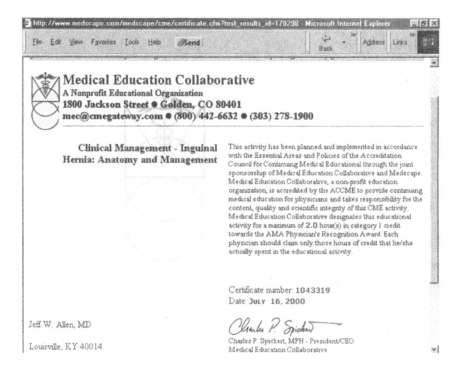

FIGURE 10.2. Instant certificate.

Examples of general surgery modules include "Inguinal Hernia: Anatomy and Management," "Update on Antithrombotic Treatment in Peripheral Arterial Disease Patients," and "Pathophysiology of Chronic Allograft Rejection." Three modules are available in urology, 13 in orthopedics, 19 in critical care, and 11 in gastroenterology.

Medscape's Web page also contains a CME conference calendar. This feature chronologically lists conferences and meetings by region and specialty that offer traditional CME. Medscape also offers a CME credit tracker. This lists the CME activities, date completed, and credit hours awarded for each registered user, and is a helpful way to keep record of this.

Helix

Healthcare Learning and Information Exchange (**http://www.helix.com**) is a Web page offering CME opportunities. It is sponsored in part by GlaxoWellcome. HELIX offers a number of services of interest to practicing physicians, nurses, and pharmacists. CME in each of these fields is available. Although not all of the programs are in the form of online modules, there are a number of opportunities to earn credit in scheduled lectures, in the teleconference home study program, and through "Healthstream University."

CME Web

CME Web (**http://www.cmeweb.com**) is the self-proclaimed "global continuing medical education resource." This site is owned by American Health Consultants and offers a larger variety of CME courses than most Web pages. However, it is a "for profit" company that charges a small fee for most of the CME. These fees are approximately $15 per credit hour. Bulk rates are available: 60 credit hours cost $300. Currently, there is no general surgery category; however a number of categories contain modules of interest to surgeons. Critical care, for example, has 37 tests with 55.5 CME credits available. There are 70.5 hours available in oncology and 4 hours in trauma.

One negative feature of CME Web is its registration process, which requires that a credit card number be entered. Many people are not entirely comfortable with E-commerce and prefer not to give out their credit card number. Fortunately, CME Web offers some courses that are free and do not require transmission of a credit card number. An example is a review and update of anticoagulation found at **http://www.vstream.com/ login/medec2/medec_login2.vhtm**.

Medconnect

The CME center of MedConnect (**http://www.medconnect.com**) is affiliated with HealthAtoZ Professional and the University of the Sciences in Philadelphia. Admission to the CME center of MedConnect requires passwords that are free with registration. Although there is no dedicated section on surgery, modules of interest to the surgeon include "Dispelling the myths: Advanced Diagnostic Imaging in Acute Appendicitis" and "Recent Advances in Rapid Sequence Intubation," which are found in the emergency medicine section.

Pain

The Web page for Pain (**http://www.pain.com**) contains an area of CME modules. Surprisingly, these modules, sponsored by Abbot Laboratories, are not entirely about pain management. Recent CME topics of interest to surgeons include "An Unusual Case of Thoracic Outlet Syndrome Associated with Long-Distance Running," "Presentation and Distribution of Antibody-Antigen Complexes in the Herniated Nucleus Pulposus," and "Assessing the Risks and Benefits of Herbal Medicine: An Overview of Scientific Evidence."

University of Washington CME

CME credit from the University of Washington CME (**http://www. uwcme.org**) requires purchase of a password. There is a one-time fee (currently $50) that allows its user to obtain an unlimited amount of credit during one year. There are some CME courses at this Web page that are free of charge and do not require a password.

Conclusion

Obtaining CME credit online is fast, easy, and inexpensive. Modules available on Web pages are generally informative, well written, and peer-reviewed. Like most Internet activities, however, obtaining online CME credit is not without imperfections. A potential abuse of the system could allow visitors to take the test without studying the material. Since the threshold for a passing grade usually is low (70%), obtaining credit with no real additional education is possible. This abuse defeats the very philosophy of CME.

11
Becoming a Presence on the Internet

Everybody's Doing It
What to Include
Production
Servers and Getting the Information to Them
Homemade Web Pages
Web Pages by Template
Conclusion

Everybody's Doing It

In the not-too-distant past, physicians who advertised their services were immediately discredited and occasionally even arrested. However, the public's attitude toward advertising of medical services has since relaxed. In fact, many medical organizations and physicians have rapidly seized the opportunity to go online. According to an American Medical Association study, over 27% of physicians in the United States have their own Web page.[1] This number is sure to grow. Creating and posting a Web page that details the services of an individual surgeon may be a form of advertising, but it also can be a valuable resource for patients, ancillary staff, and referring physicians. Potential benefits to the physician who has a personal Web page include better-informed patients, simplified communications, and increased referrals.

What to Include

A physician's Web page has the potential to be more than an accepted form of personal advertising. A section on "Frequently Asked Questions" (FAQs) may preempt and answer patients' common inquiries. A section on "What to Watch for" with a description of postoperative conditions and examples for early diagnosis may prompt patients to seek medical advice early rather than late. Other helpful details include directions to the medical facility, a listing of office hours, and how to refill prescriptions (Table 11.1).

TABLE 11.1. Top ten items to be included in a personal physician Web site.

 1. Office phone number and after-hours number
 2. Hours of operation
 3. Driving directions to the office as well as to hospitals used by the physician
 4. E-mail address
 5. Insurance and health plans accepted
 6. Privacy statement
 7. Photograph and professional credentials in a CV format
 8. Frequently asked questions
 9. List of the diagnoses commonly treated by the physician
10. Patient information section

Production

The first hurdle in the production of a Web page involves interest on the part of the physician. The second hurdle involves the actual creation of the Web page. There are a number of ways that a surgeon can achieve both and "hang" a shingle in cyberspace. One is to continue reading about the subject, and another is to begin to design your own Web page.

Many expensive and aesthetically pleasing Web pages are professionally designed (Figure 11.1). This entails hiring a Web page design company. These companies employ graphic artists, text authors, and computer programmers. Depending on their expertise and familiarity with medicine and surgery, these professionals may have good ideas for a Web page. However, the physician should write the text. The notion of relying on your design company to write you "top 10 reasons to have breast augmentation" is far-fetched. Instead, provide the company with all of the text, images (with written permission from identifiable subjects, if needed), and your curriculum vitae. Be aware that hiring design professionals is expensive. Although prices vary, a ballpark figure is $5,000. If a professional Web page is provided for less, consider yourself lucky. If the professional charges more, do not be surprised. Initial Web page design alone has cost as much as $100,000 for the impressive and elaborate pages that use the maximum number of "bells and whistles."

Unfortunately, the creation of a Web page is only half the challenge. Once the company you hire has finished the design and you have approved it, you most likely will receive a floppy disk containing the files of your Web page. The information on this disk must be sent online to a server. (This disk has a tendency to be carried around in a briefcase for a couple of weeks and may ultimately be lost. This is a far cry from the millions of visitors you were expecting and the e-mailboxes stuffed with consultations.)

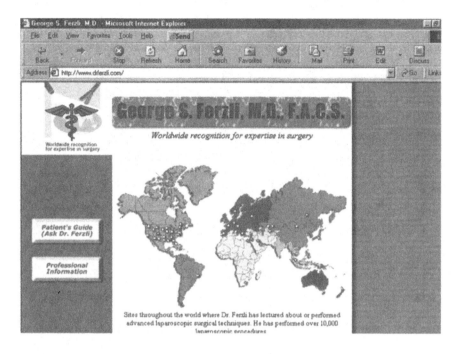

FIGURE 11.1. The Web page for Dr. Ferzli was professionally created. (Reprinted with permission from George Ferzli, MD.)

Servers and Getting the Information to Them

A server basically is an Internet-based computer program, administered by a private company, that displays your Web page when other computers call on it. (This is called domain hosting.) A server also is a storage place for your Web page files and, of course, entails a cost. Ordinary charges for domain hosting services are approximately $30 per month, but they may be much more depending on the size of your Web page. Many universities will allow its faculty access to a server for free or at a discounted rate. Some Internet Service Providers, like America Online, will provide server space to its customers for their personal Web pages; however, this use is often restricted to exclude any commercial content.

A File Transfer Protocol (FTP) program also is needed to transfer your material from a computer (or the disk that contains the Web page files) to the server. Some Web page companies will offer the service of "FTPing" your Web page files to your server (Figure 11.2).

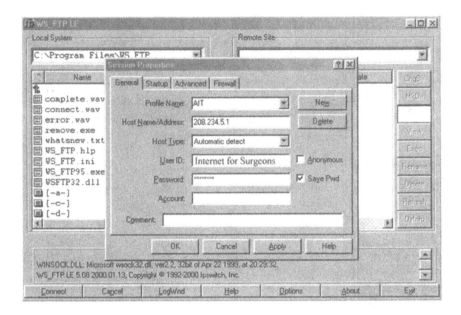

FIGURE 11.2. WS FTP LE in action. (Reprinted with permission from Arthur L. Beal.)

Homemade Web Pages

If the above sounds a bit excessive for your modest project, you are not alone. Indeed, most of the physician Web pages online today are not professionally produced. An obvious option is to create the Web page yourself. This requires a bit of knowledge, motivation, persistence, and software. A Hypertext Markup Language (HTML) editor is the program needed to create a Web page. It is similar to a word processor, and often it is as easy (and sometimes as difficult) to use. HTML editors may be purchased for as little as $30. A free HTML editor is available from America Online. This product is called "AOLpress," and it is "freeware" that can be downloaded from the Web page at **http://www.aolpress.com**. This HTML editor does not require that the resultant Web page be hosted with American Online.

One of the most common word processors is Microsoft Word, and it is available on many IBM-class computers. Word documents may be converted to Web page language, and thus this word processor works as an HTML editor. To use Word in this way, type in a document in Word and then choose the option "Save as Web Page." One problem with this technique is that it is difficult to go back and edit a Web page created using Word.

If your self-made Web page is to contain graphics, software such as Jasc Paintshop Pro or Adope Photoshop will be helpful. Demonstration copies may be downloaded from Jasc (**http://www.jasc.com**) or Adobe (**http://www.adobe.com**). The types of graphic files that Web browsers are able to recognize and display contain the suffixes ".gif" or ".jpeg." These are referred to as gifs (g pronounced as in gypsy) and j-pegs, respectively. Microsoft Paint, a built-in feature of many IBM-class computers, also may be used to create and manipulate gifs. Microsoft Paint is available under the accessories of the Windows heading.

After creation of a personal Web page, the Web page files will be stored on a hard drive or disk (e.g., a briefcase), but are not available for public viewing yet. To move your files to your server, a File Transfer Protocol (FTP) program is necessary. To use the FTP program, a host name or address, user identification, and password are required. This information is readily available from your domain host company. A freely downloaded FTP program, WS-FTP LE, is available to many qualified users from its designer's Web page at **http://www.ipswitch.com**.

Web Pages by Template

If you do not want to pay a large sum of money for your Web page or learn the skills necessary to create a Web page, there is another, even simpler way to stake a claim to a piece of the information superhighway for yourself. Many of the large, corporate medical Web pages, such as Medscape (**http://www.medscape.com**) and WebMD (**http://www.webmd. com**), offer member physicians the opportunity to easily create and publish a Web page. Some medical societies are beginning to offer this service as well. Creation of a Web page using a template can be accomplished free of charge and is done entirely by way of an online fill-in-the-blanks system.

Interested physicians can sign up with Medscape, for example, and then choose "Create or Edit my Web Page" from the left-sided menu on the Medscape homepage (**http://www.medscape.com**). First, select a color scheme and an image for a logo. Next, enter office hours, location, after-hours contact for emergencies, credentials, special interests or experiences, and hospital or health plan information. Data about the members of the physician's group and additional, more personalized information also may be included.

Internet-savvy surgeons can complete such forms in less than 30 minutes. The resultant Web page is automatically posted on the Web. This conveniently bypasses the FTP step altogether. The URL for the created

Web page is **http://doctor.medscape.com/yourname**. An example of a Web page that I completed is available at **http://doctor.medscape. com/JeffAllenMD** (Figure 11.3).

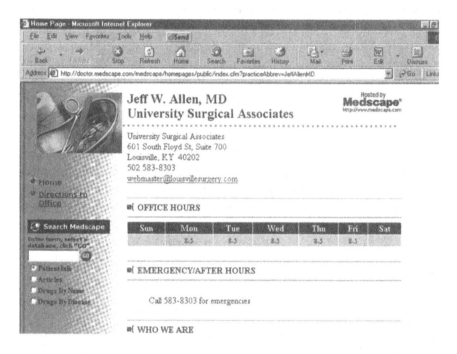

FIGURE 11.3. Medscape-created Web page for the author. (Reprinted with permission from Hiram C. Polk, Jr., MD, University Surgical Associates.)

The benefits of the template approach include the low (or no) cost and ease of inputting information, and that there is no need for a server. The Medscape-, WebMD-, or other template-created Web pages can be linked to and registered with search engines, just like the professionally created pages. The main drawbacks to using these templates include a perceived affiliation with the corporation and the relative inflexibility of the templates themselves.

Conclusion

Options available to the surgeon who wants a personal Web page are summarized in Table 11.2. Higher budget projects are usually completed by a professional Web page design company. Although this is a costly approach, the Web pages often have a refined, polished appearance, and the

TABLE 11.2. Comparing features of different types of Web pages.

Web page production approach	Ease of creation	Cost	Quality of appearance	Level of knowledge required	Need for server	Ease of updating	Constraints on design
Professional	Medium	High	High	Medium	Yes	Low	None
Template	High	None	Low	Low/none	No	High	High
Self-made	Low	Low/None	Variable	High	Yes	Low	Low/none

surgeon is spared having to learn about the inner workings of a Web page. Do-it-yourselfers may learn the HTML and use HTML editors and graphics programs to create their own Web page. Novices to Web page design can use templates from corporations such as Medscape to establish a free Web page. There are significant and inflexible design constraints with this method, but the project is free of charge.

Reference

1. *American Medical News* April 24, 2000;20–21.

12
Web Page Resources by Surgical Specialty

Bariatric Surgery
Cardiac and Thoracic Surgery
Colorectal Surgery
General Surgery
Genitourinary Surgery
Hand Surgery
Minimal Access Surgery
Neurosurgery
Orthopedic Surgery
Otolaryngologic Surgery
Pediatric Surgery
Plastic and Reconstructive Surgery
Transplant Surgery
Trauma Surgery
Vascular Surgery
General Surgery Products

The Web pages cited here have been visited recently, and verification has been made prior to publication that the Web pages were up and running. Like any commercial venture, however, some of these sites may no longer be in business.

Bariatric Surgery

American Society for Bariatric Surgery (http://www.asbs.org)

Founded in 1983, the American Society for Bariatric Surgery publicizes the art and science of surgery for the morbidly obese. Visitors can calculate their body mass index (BMI) by typing in their height in feet and

inches and their weight in pounds. A membership listing by state provides the names and office telephone numbers of surgeons who specialize in treating morbidly obese patients. Also available on this Web site is
information about upcoming society meetings, a newsletter in Adobe Acrobat format, and a history of the specialty. A comprehensive section on
the rationale for the surgical treatment of severe obesity is included.

Association for Morbid Obesity Support (http://www.obesityhelp.com/morbidobesity)

This site offers peer support for patients considering surgery for obesity.
The information presented is timely, well organized, and generally helpful. A section written by patients covers the sagas of insurance hassles
and gives a fairly clear indication of which insurers typically approve
bariatric procedures. A list of members of the association who have undergone surgery is available and includes their BMI, e-mail address, in-
surer, and surgeon. Often, patients' before and after data are presented,
and photographs are included (see Figure 12.1) for the association's Web
page.

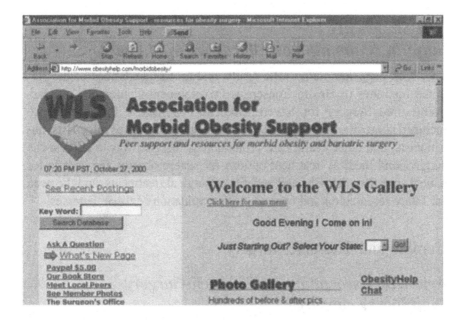

FIGURE 12.1. The Web page for the Association for Morbid Obesity Support.

BioEnterics (*http://www.bioenterics.com*)

This small company, a division of InaMed, develops and produces silicone and fiberoptic devices. Its products include two devices used in the surgical treatment of morbid obesity, the LAP-BAND adjustable gastric banding system, and the intragastric balloon system. Although neither device is currently available for widespread distribution in the United States, Food and Drug Administration approval for the LAP-BAND is expected soon. Outside the United States, the LAP-BAND has become widely used in surgery for morbid obesity. It has been used since 1993 in Europe, Canada, Australia, Mexico, Asia, Israel, and other countries. Check this Web page for updates on the status of its use in the United States.

International Federation for the Surgery of Obesity (*http://www.obesity-online.com/ifsol/*)

This organization guides surgeons interested in or already engaged in the practice of bariatric surgery. A statement is placed on the Web page to help surgeons understand what qualifications are considered acceptable to the international community of bariatric surgeons. A comprehensive meeting schedule is available as well as a list of surgeons throughout the world who routinely perform bariatric operations.

NIH Statement (*http://text.nlm.nih.gov/nih/cdc/www/84.html*)

This Web page summarizes the results and recommendations of the National Institutes of Health Consensus Development Conference on Gastrointestinal Surgery for Severe Obesity. Panelists at that conference included surgeons, gastroenterologists, endocrinologists, psychiatrists, nutritionists, and other health care professionals. Its goal was to address the surgical and medical treatment options for severe obesity, the criteria for patient selection, the risks and benefits of surgical treatments, and the need for future research on and epidemiologic evaluation of these therapies.

Cardiac and Thoracic Surgery

American Association for Thoracic Surgery (*http://www.aats.org*)

This large Web page contains a listing of members and events; a link to the association's journal, *The Journal of Thoracic and Cardiovascular*

Surgery (http://jtcs.ctsnetjournals.org) (Figure 12.2); case presentations; and the activities of the numerous committees of the association. An annual report is included, with contributions from each of the committees and from representatives to other organizations, such as the American Association of Blood Banks and the National Association for Biomedical Research. Also available is information about applications for grants, fellowships, and scholarships, including the American Association for Thoracic Surgery Evarts A. Graham Memorial Traveling Fellowship, the John H. Gibbon, Jr., Research Scholarship, and an International Traveling Fellowship.

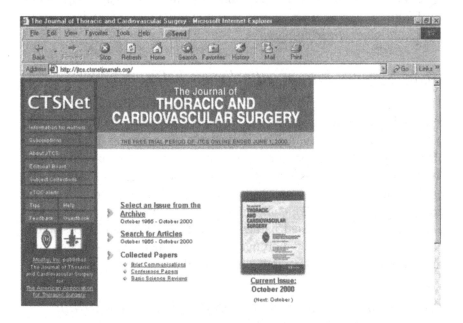

FIGURE 12.2. The online *Journal of Thoracic and Cardiovascular Surgery.*

American Heart Association
(http://www.americanheart.org)

The American Heart Association is dedicated to providing the public with information on fighting heart disease and stroke. For the health care professional, a section offering continuing medical education credit is available. Well-made slides are available for lecture topics such as "Guidelines for Perioperative Cardiovascular Evaluation for Noncardiac Surgery" and "Genome-Based Resource for Molecular Cardiovascular

Medicine: Toward a Compendium of Cardiovascular Genes." There are in PowerPoint format, and the entire presentations may be downloaded to a personal computer for future use as a slide show.

Cardiothoracic Surgery Network (http://www.ctsnet.org)

This frequently updated comprehensive site has many highlights. One area details controversies in cardiothoracic surgery and contains extensive discussions, in debate form, among leading experts in the field. The Power Point slide presentations used by debaters are included, and the audio (in Real Audio format) often is available. Also included on the Cardiothoracic Surgery Network's Web page are photo and video galleries, a product forum, a clinical trials section, job opportunities, and reviews about other cardiothoracic Web pages.

Heart Surgery Forum (http://www.hsforum.com)

This Web page is a cardiothoracic multimedia journal and is edited by Dr. Mark Levinson. It currently is sponsored by Genzyme (**http://www. genzyme.com**). Visitors may view abstracts of upcoming meetings. The Heart Surgery Forum sponsors several unique automated e-mail forums for discussing various aspects of clinical practice in cardiac surgery. Included are open heart, closed heart, minimally invasive direct coronary artery bypass (MIDCAB), congenital, and chest listsevers. A jobs board is displayed, and interested parties may list their availability or inquire about a currently posted opportunity for employment. This site also publishes original investigative and clinical work.

International Society for Minimally Invasive Cardiac Surgery (http://www.ismics.org)

Formed in 1997 by the participants of the World Congress of Minimally Invasive Cardiac Surgery, this organization has a leadership role in less invasive methods of performing cardiac surgery. This site features online submission of abstracts for its scientific meeting. Archived abstracts of previous meetings are available. Board members, upcoming meetings, and bylaws also are described.

Society of Thoracic Surgeons (http://www.STS.org)

This national data bank lists cardiothoracic procedures accrued yearly from over 500 participating centers. Statistics are available for over 1.3

million cardiac procedures. Length of stay, mortality rates, and risk-adjusted mortality rates are discussed. A "For Patients" area describes what a thoracic surgeon is and explains the diagnosis and treatment of common diseases of the chest.

Thoracic Surgery Foundation for Research and Education (http://www.tsfre.org)

This society was founded to "enhance the education and capabilities of thoracic surgeons for tomorrow." Numerous grants, research awards, and scholarships funded by philanthropy are available from this society for young investigators in the field of cardiothoracic surgery. The application process is explained online, as are the specifics of the available grants. Tax-deductible donations to the foundation are solicited.

Colorectal Surgery

American Society of Colon and Rectal Surgeons (http://www.fascrs.org)

This is one of the leading colorectal professional organizations and represents over 1,000 surgeons. More than 20 online patient brochures are available from this Web page. These cover subjects such as "What Is an Ostomy?"; "Screening and Surveillance for Colorectal Cancer"; and "New Surgical Options for the Treatment of Ulcerative Colitis." A special section enables visitors to locate a colorectal surgeon in their area. The page details practice parameters on subjects from ambulatory anorectal surgery to sigmoid diverticulitis. An online calendar lists events of interest to the colorectal surgeon.

Colorectal Cancer Screening (http://www.gastro.org/colcancer/)

This Web page is a section of the larger page for the American Gastroenterological Association (**http://www.gastro.org**). It contains the findings and recommendations of an independent expert panel studying screening programs for colorectal cancer. Panelists included consumers, oncologists, colorectal surgeons, economists, and gastroenterologists. Introductory subjects, such as the adenoma-carcinoma sequence, are described and provide insight into the group's final recommendations for screening frequency and method.

Crohn's and Colitis Foundation of America (http://www.ccfa.org)

The goal of this society is to eliminate Crohn's disease and ulcerative colitis. A physician's resource room is designed for health care professionals who frequently treat inflammatory bowel disease. Articles about the various aspects of inflammatory bowel disease, including treatment guidelines, are located here. A calendar of events lists upcoming meetings of interest to physicians treating Crohn's disease and ulcerative colitis. Brochures designed for patients also are available.

Digestive Disease Week (http://www.ddw.org)

Online registration and a complete calendar of events are available for this conference, which is rapidly becoming one of the largest in the world. Guidelines for oral presentations and posters are included as is housing and travel accommodation information. A Digestive Disease Week electronic job placement service is available on this Web page. A meeting planner/abstract search can help maximize attendance of visitors to the sessions of their choice.

Society for Surgery of the Alimentary Tract (http://www.ssat.com)

The area of this Web page most likely to be visited by health care professionals is entitled "Guidelines for Physicians." Here, the recommendations of the society on topics such as the surgical management of diverticulitis are published. According to the Web page, these guidelines are intended for primary care doctors. In many instances, these sections are available in English, Spanish, and Japanese. Also included on the society's Web page are a list of members, an application for membership, a link to the *Journal of GI Surgery*, and abstracts from the previous Digestive Week conferences.

United Ostomy Association (http://www.uoa.org)

This association is a support group for patients with stomas. A proactive organization, it has lobbied for legislation requiring insurance companies to pay for early screening tests for colon cancer. An online form used to join the society can be printed out and mailed in. Books and merchandise are sold on the Web page to help support the association. One of the sponsors of the Web page is G.G.'s Dignity Wear, Inc. (**http://www.ggsdignity.**

com), a company that specializes in garments for patients with ostomies or urologic appliances (Figure 12.3).

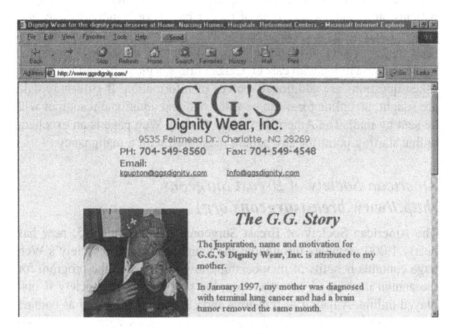

FIGURE 12.3. The Web page for G.G.'s Dignity Wear, Inc. (Reprinted with permission from Kenneth A. Gupton.)

General Surgery

American Board of Surgery (http://www.absurgery.org)

Founded in 1937, the American Board of Surgery (ABS) recognizes those surgeons who meet specific academic requirements and complete a series of examinations. The ABS is an independent, nonprofit organization and is one of the 24 certifying boards that are members of the American Board of Medical Specialties. The Web page for the ABS includes the purpose of the board, examinations offered, the dates and application deadlines for the exams, and the requirement for admission and certification. Information about credit for foreign graduate education also is available on-line. Inquiries as to surgeon certification status are addressed; the policy of the ABS, as explained on the Web page, is to answer written and telephone inquiries about the board certification status of a surgeon directly. Recertification, currently considered voluntary, also is discussed on this Web page.

American Cancer Society (*http://www.cancer.org*)

The American Cancer Society (ACS) slogan, "Hope, Progress, Answers," is proudly displayed on this Web page. The site is directed primarily to patients, and nearly every type of cancer has its own individual section online. Each of these cancer-specific Web pages includes discussions of such topics as what it is, prevention, risk factors, detection, symptoms, treatment, and living with cancer. Cancer drugs, a glossary, and frequently asked questions are additional sources of information. If still more data are sought, an online form can be filled out, and additional resources will be sent by mail. The American Cancer Society Web page is an excellent online starting point for any patient diagnosed with a malignancy.

American Society of Breast Surgeons (*http://www.breastsurgeons.org*)

The American Society of Breast Surgeons, founded in 1995, now has nearly 1,000 members throughout the United States. The society's Web page contains benefits of membership, how to join, and the program for the annual meeting. A message from the president of the society is displayed online. A listing of registries and clinical trials as well as contact information for those studies are included. Consensus statements, including the guidelines for sentinel lymph node biopsy, are available.

Association of Academic Surgical Administrators (*http://www.aasagroup.org*)

The Association of Academic Surgical Administrators (AASA), founded in 1983, has grown from a group of 50 charter members to over 165 surgeons representing 80 academic surgical practices in 38 states, the District of Columbia, and Canada. The AASA promotes opportunities for the academic surgeon in the U.S. today. Included on this Web page is "The Cutting Edge," the AASA's newsletter. A list of links of interest to the academic surgeon is available, along with a guideline for recruiting surgery administrators. An AASA roster with contact information including e-mail addresses is displayed.

Association of Women Surgeons (*http://www.womensurgeons.org*)

The Association of Women Surgeons (AWS), founded in 1981, uses its Web page to highlight the *Pocket Mentor*, a manual for surgical interns and residents written in 1994 by AWS member Joyce A. Majure, M.D. This book was designed to help surgeons in training and is based on the experience of a number of women surgeons. An AWS 2000 version of the *Pocket Mentor* is expected. A twice-yearly conference is detailed on the Web page, and online discussion groups are available. Membership in the organization is offered to female physicians holding the M.D. or D.O. degrees (or their international equivalents) and who are considered surgeons. A membership application request form is available from this Web page.

Fellowship of the American College of Surgeons (*http://www.facs.org*)

The Web page for the American College of Surgeons (ACS) is one of the most extensive sites on the Internet with a focus on surgery (Figure 12.4). Among the many highlights are the Surgical Education Self-Assessment Program (SESAP) sample questions. High-definition radiographs, computed tomography (CT) scans, and other visual aids are included with the multiple-choice questions and fully annotated answers. A running tally of the questions answered correctly is kept automatically. A "Career Opportunities and Position Résumé Data Bank" is available, but access is restricted to members of the ACS. Many of the state chapters of the ACS have a Web page, and a list of links to these chapters is avail-

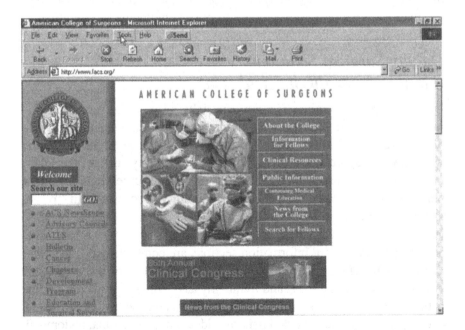

FIGURE 12.4. The Web page for the American College of Surgeons. (Reprinted with permission from Linn Meyer.)

able. A list of ways to obtain continuing medical education credit is included on this comprehensive Web page.

General Surgery Patient Information
(http://www.Internets.com/mednets/gensurgpat.htm)

This general surgery section from Mednets is an excellent links page, but contains little else. Clinical information, such as stomach and liver anatomy, and an online laparoscopic technical manual are available by way of links from this Web page. Although many of the links are geared toward patient education, a number of pages are aimed at general surgeons. Subjects covered include treatment of gallstones, tumor markers, wound care, and antibiotic prophylaxis.

Internal Museum of Surgical Science
(http://www.imss.org)

An interactive antique illness section puts you in your forefather's shoes, diagnosing an illness such as a bladder stone with treatments like bloodletting, magnesium sulfate, and the use of a lithotrite. This Web page represents the actual museum, located in Chicago and displaying exhibits on over 4,000 years of surgery. Information includes school tour availability, internship opportunities, admission prices, and hours of operation.

Quality Surgical Solutions
(http://www.qualitysurgical.com)

Quality Surgical Solutions is a multispecialty group of surgeons in Kentucky and southern Indiana who partnered with local hospitals and national insurance firms to study and improve the quality of surgical care while decreasing cost. On their Web page, a monthly feature, the Pharmacy Corner, discusses different aspects of general surgery and the pharmacology of associated drug therapy. In addition, excerpts from "When to Refer to a Specialist: A Gatekeeper's Manual" are available on subjects such as gastrointestinal bleeding, myringotomy tubes, and melanoma. The patient information sections are comprehensive and contain an introduction about the normal organ, disorders of the organ, the procedure, before and after, and frequently asked questions. Topics in the patient information section (Figure 12.5) cover colonoscopy, laparoscopic cholecystectomy, radio-guided parathyroidectomy, melanoma, abdominal aortic aneurysm repair, and appendectomy, among many others.

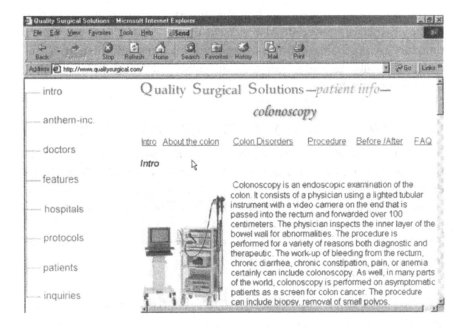

FIGURE 12.5. Patient information from Quality Surgical Solutions. (Reprinted with permission from Kenneth J. DeSimone, MD, Quality Surgical Solutions.)

Genitourinary Surgery

American Foundation for Urologic Disease (http://www.afud.org/home.html)

The American Foundation for Urologic Disease answers over 5,000 calls from patients per month on its toll-free information network and earmarks over $2.4 million in urology research and public education initiatives. Highlighting this organization's Web page is the "Prostate Cancer Resource Guide." This includes an overview of the physiology of the normal and abnormal prostate gland, pharmacology of treating prostate cancer, and treatment options. Also available from the Foundation's Web page is patient-directed information about overactive bladders and incontinence.

American Urologic Association (http://www.auanet.org)

Among many of the high spots of the Web page for the American Urologic Association (AUA) is the William P. Didusch Museum. The museum is a past and present look at a collection of urologic instruments, topics, and books. Subjects such as the history of transurethral resection of the prostate are covered. Also present on the AUA's Web page are a directory of practicing members, upcoming meeting information, a calendar of events, and information for news media. A link to URomart is prominently displayed.

Contemporary Urology (*http://www.conturo.com*)

A monthly publication sponsored by *Medical Economics*, this site focuses on practical reviews and updates in genitourinary surgery. Topics covered include infertility, incontinence, erectile dysfunction, and oncology. On occasion, pediatrics, female urology, and infectious diseases are explored. An index of articles is arranged by topic and is comprehensive. The "conference center" allows urologists to chat online with their colleagues about specific subjects.

Digital Urology Journal (*http://www.duj.com/*)

The *Digital Urology Journal* is an online, peer-reviewed journal of adult and pediatric urology, sponsored in part by Boston Scientific Microinvasive (Figure 12.6). Some of the most educational areas of this site are the

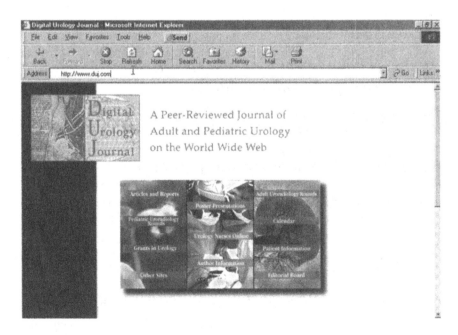

FIGURE 12.6. The Web page for the *Digital Urology Journal*. (Reprinted with permission from Anthony Atala, MD.)

adult and pediatric uroradiology rounds sections. These contain CT scans, radiographs, intravenous pylograms, and magnetic resonance images from cases at the Brigham and Women's Hospital of the Harvard Medical School. These are in the form of case studies and include the diagnosis and discussion of the problem and the pertinence of the tests. Sixty-seven grants in urologic research are available from this Web page, and the applications, in most instances, are included.

Society for Pediatric Urology (http://www.spu.org)

The Society for Pediatric Urology Web page contains a "Find a Pediatric Urologist" function that allows users to find names of members in their state. A mailing list is available from the Web page. The goals of this list are outlined on the page and include discussing clinical problems with colleagues, promoting research, and disseminating information to members. The John W. Duckett, Jr., Research Scholarship is available from the society, and information about it is available online.

Urology News (http://www.uroreviews.org)

This Web page is a bimonthly review of the current literature in genitourinary surgery. Urology News displays articles and features areas of current interest, important conference reviews, and product information important to the practicing urologist. Registration is free, and members may be asked to complete online product surveys. These surveys often offer compensation (up to $100). During registration, applicants are asked if they would like to be notified when the Web page for Urology News is updated.

Uronet (http://www.uronet.org/index.html)

Admission to the Uronet Web page requires a password, which can be obtained through a free registration process. In "Current Controversies," an open-forum discussion takes place online in which practicing urologists and other health care professionals express their opinions about controversial urologic problems. In "Diary Dates," upcoming scientific meetings are listed in chronological order, with Web page and e-mail links included where available. "URO Challenge" is a test segment of the page, consisting of ten multiple choice questions that are marked electronically.

Uroreviews (http://www.uroreviews.org)

Uroreviews is a Web page that is written by urologists for urologists and associated specialists. It provides up-to-the-minute reviews of topics in the urologic literature. The reviews typically condense the journal articles and critically discuss the conclusions that may be drawn based on the article. A search function makes it easier to find an exact topic of interest.

Hand Surgery

American Association for Hand Surgery (http://www.handsurgery.org)

Research awards, established to "foster creativity and innovation" in hand surgery, are available from the American Association for Hand Surgery to residents, fellows, and therapists. An application form is provided at this Web site, but it must be mailed in after completion. Nominations also may be made for the Vargas International Hand Therapist Award, named in honor of Dr. Miguel Vargas. A calendar of events and conference information are obtainable on this site.

American Society for Surgery of the Hand (http://www.hand-surg.org)

This organization provides continuing medical education through meetings, seminars, online skills, self-assessment programs, and publications about the hand and upper extremity. A listing of international meetings on hand surgery is included, along with contact information for those meetings. Often, the meetings have their own Web page, and those are duly linked here. A book and a video library are cataloged online. The public information section contains a "Find-a-Doc" section that lists (by state and name) surgeons in a local area with a specific interest in surgery of the hand.

e-Hand, Electronic Textbook of Hand Surgery (http://www.eatonhand.com)

Handling over 27,000 hits per day, this is surely one of the busiest of the hand surgery Web sites. Visitors may view the anatomy of the hand in great detail through online images on this Web page. Although the taxonomy system that navigates the site can be difficult to use, the resulting graphics files (referenced to Primal Pictures) are quite well made and instructional. The "Handbase" case of the week archives contains two years of monthly cases with high-quality images of radiographs and good discussions.

Hand Transplant (*http://www.handtransplant.com*)

Matthew Scott, recipient of the first hand transplant performed in the United States, takes center stage in this Web page (Figure 12.7). Having lost his dominant hand in 1985 in a fireworks explosion, he underwent the transplant in January 1999. Intraoperative photographs are available as well as an impressive picture of Scott using his transplanted hand to throw out the first pitch before the Philadelphia Phillies' opening game just three months after the surgery. Future possible recipients can learn more basic facts online and may seek additional information by e-mail.

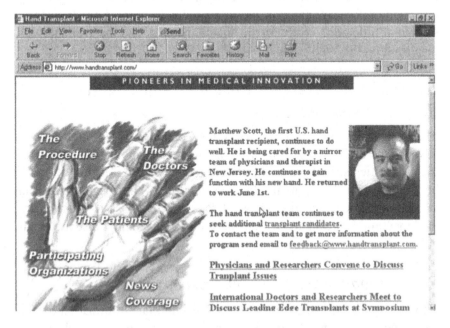

FIGURE 12.7. The Web page for Hand Transplant. (Reprinted with permission from Barbara S. Mackovic.)

International Hand Library (http://www.handlibrary.org)

An official repository for documents of the International Federation of Societies for Surgery of the Hand, this Web page contains a calendar of events including contact information for each event. The vendor market-place section is a comprehensive list of the products and services of interest to hand surgeons. Members of the organization can gain access to additional, exclusive areas of the Web site. Cases may be submitted for discussion in some sections.

Minimal Access Surgery

European Association for Endoscopic Surgery (http://www.europeanaes.org)

The society with the most interest in evidence-based laparoscopic surgery is the European Association for Endoscopic Surgery (EAES). *Surgical Endoscopy*, the official journal of this organization, is included as a link. Also available are instructions for applying for membership and meeting information. Educational courses for surgeons in training are frequently offered at little or no cost with the annual meeting, and the availability is displayed on the Web page.

International Society for Computer Aided Surgery (http://www.iscas.org)

The goal of the International Society for Computer Aided Surgery is to advance the utilization of computers and related technologies in the treatment of patients. Visitors to the Web page may view a listing of members along with their e-mail addresses. Those seeking membership can fill out an online application. A list of society activities, including the annual meeting, is included. Sections on statutes and counsel also are available.

Laparoscopy (http://www.laparoscopy.com)

This multiple award–winning Web site has important information for the laparoscopist or general surgeon practicing laparoscopy. The video and picture galleries are outstanding and provide a way to learn key parts of complex procedures online. The site makes physician referrals to patients who need surgery, based on the laparoscopic database. To be listed in the referral base, simply fill in the online form. This Web site provides an interactive look at the advancing technology of laparoscopic surgery and other microinvasive techniques.

Laparoscopy.net (http://www.laparoscopy.net)

Originating from the St. Joseph's Medical Center in Burbank, California, this Web page details many of the technical points in laparoscopic surgery. This site includes excerpts from the book *Interventional Laparoscopy, The State of the Art for the New Millennium* by Dr. Philippe J. Quilici. Many of the topics, which are grouped by procedure (such as laparoscopic inguinal hernia repair or laparoscopic common bile duct exploration), contain diagrams and illustrations. These include operating room setup, basic anatomy, and operative technique. More complex procedures, such as laparoscopic Nissen fundoplication with lengthening gastroplasty, are included. This is one of the best online laparoscopic atlases.

Pediatric Laparoscopy (http://www.geocities.com/~endopediatric)

This site includes a photo gallery that has intraoperative images of pediatric surgical problems such as intussusception and Meckel's diverticulum. The *Journal of Pediatric Laparoscopy* may be viewed here as well. Links to books about pediatric laparoscopy are listed with ordering information from the large online bookstore, Amazon.com (**http://www. amazon.com**).

Society of American Gastrointestinal Endoscopic Surgeons (http://www.sages.org)

The Web page for the largest endoscopic surgery organization in the world does not disappoint. This page contains meeting information, online abstract submission, publications, and a job board. The slide show quizzes are well done but do display the scores of the surgeons who have tested their luck with them. Since not all of the quizzes contain answers that are universally accepted as fact by all general surgeons, this can be an aggravating section of the Web page. A reminder service alerts (by way of e-mail) those who sign up with the service when a new set of slide quizzes has been placed online. Recently, an audio presentation of the lecture series has been added. The most exciting area of this Web page is the outcomes project, an ambitious venture that will examine the results of laparoscopic surgical procedure by each individual surgeon.

Society of Laparoendoscopic Surgeons (http://www.sls.org)

Explanation of the benefits of membership in the Society of Laparoendoscopic Surgeons (SLS) highlight this concise Web page. Members are listed by state and specialty and serve as a referral for patients who might happen onto the site. Meeting information is included for the SLS as well as other similar organizations. The organization's publication, the *Journal of the Society of Laparoendoscopic Surgeons*, is under construction here; however, guidelines for authors may be viewed. Under the resident section, a program called Mentor Match is described. This was developed by the society to help match experienced laparoscopic surgeons with residents or less experienced surgeons wishing to further their knowledge and skills in minimal access surgical techniques. A discussion group listserver is available.

Neurosurgery

Acute Stroke Toolbox (http://www.stroke-site.org)

The Acute Stroke Toolbox is a links page designed for health care professionals who develop systems for rapid diagnosis and management for patients with acute or evolving strokes. It includes links to guidelines from the American Heart Association for thrombolytic therapy for acute stroke, management of patients with acute ischemic stroke, and management of aneurysmal subarachnoid hemorrhages. There also are resources such as the Stroke Coding Guide of the American Academy of Neurology. Links to pathways for treatment also are available. This Web page is well organized and easy to follow.

American Brain Tumor Association (http://www.abta.org)

Included on this extensive Web page is a primer of brain tumors, the patient's reference manual. This online booklet was written to help patients and their families learn about and better understand malignancies affecting the brain. It includes anatomic parts of the brain, brain tumor basics, and symptoms to watch for. A "Facts and Statistics" section describes the incidence and trends in diagnosing and treating brain cancers. The statistics for pediatric patients also are included because brain tumors are the second leading cause of cancer-related deaths in patients under the age of 20. (Leukemia remains the first.) A "Comfort and Resources" section of this Web page details numerous patients with both favorable and unfavorable outcomes and is a realistic source for patient resources. An area for health care professionals who treat brain cancers includes links to journals, a descriptive listing of available research funding, an international meeting calendar, patient education tools, and description and links to several national clinical trial databases.

Brain Tumor Society (*http://www.tbts.org*)

The primary mission of the Brain Tumor Society (BTS) is to promote ways to find a cure for brain tumors and to improve the quality of life of those patients with brain tumors. This Web page often is in outline form but includes basic information about brain tumors, patient and family resources, an online newsletter, and a frequently asked questions section. Resources for health care providers include a guide to brain tumors for the primary care physician. Funding for basic science research projects in this area is sponsored by the BTS and is available at a maximum of $50,000 per year for each approved project. An "Events and Conferences" schedule, links section, and brain tumor booklists complete the Web page.

Clinical Trials and Noteworthy Treatments for Brain Tumors (*http://www.virtualtrials.com*)

This Web page, sponsored in part by Rhône-Poulenc-Rorer, is maintained by the Musella Foundation for Brain Tumor Research. It consists of a database of treatment for brain tumors. Begun in 1993 as a text file, it has since been expanded into a Web site. The data included within the Web page are obtained by surveying the major institutions that treat brain cancers around the world. The database is searchable as well as grouped by treatment modality, including radiation, chemotherapy, immunotherapy, and surgical trials.

Facial Neuralgia Resources (*http://facial-neuralgia.org*)

This Web page includes resources on the conditions of facial neuralgia, other cranial neuralgias, dental conditions, and neuralgia-like disorders (Figure 12.8). Drugs, surgery, and alternative treatments are discussed on this Web page. Medicine is described, e.g., dosages, possible side effects, medical references, and positive, mixed, and negative patient experiences. Lingering questions such as drug treatment versus surgery, dosage levels, and blood tests also are discussed. Sections on support, coping skills,

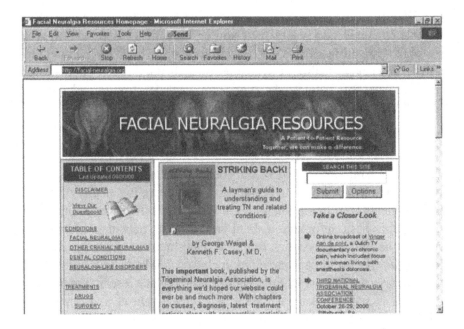

FIGURE 12.8. The Web page for Facial Neuralgia Resources. (Reprinted with permission from Leslie Carroll, Facial Neuralgia Resources.)

and research are available. Live international chats with experts in the field are highlighted on this Web page. An online report of the 1998 Trigeminal Neuralgia Association International Conference is available, as are links to clinical trials for oral facial neuralgias.

Hydrocephalus Association (*http://www.hydroassoc.org*)

Individual contributors, membership dues, grants from private corporations and foundations, and a yearly fund-raising drive fund the Hydrocephalus Association. The services of this organization include an outreach program that provides free information and resources to patients and their families, a telephone support system that provides one-to-one counseling, social gatherings, networking with support groups, and a variety of scholarships and prizes. Included in the latter is the Gerald S. Fudge Scholarship, created in 1993, which recognizes accomplishments of young adults with hydrocephalus and helps to fund college and graduate education for patients afflicted with hydrocephalus. In addition, an annual prize is given by the association for the best research paper on hydrocephalus presented that year by a neurosurgical resident. The "Hydrocephalus Fact Sheet" provides basic scientific information about the condition as well as hospitalization tips and a description of a third ventriculostomy, billed as a promising procedure of the future.

Neurosurgery On Call (http://www.aans.org)

This Web page includes the popular features "Find a Neurosurgeon" and "Ask a Neurosurgeon." "Ask a Neurosurgeon" enables patients, health care professionals, and interested parties to submit questions via e-mail, which are then individually answered. There also are resources pages for herniated disks, head injury, epilepsy, stroke, carpal tunnel syndrome, and many other conditions. The search function allows you to find a neurosurgeon based on area code, last name, city and state, or country. An "In the News" section, updated weekly, includes headlines and complete stories about neurosurgical topics in the press today. Patient resources include instructive online pamphlets about topics such as anatomy of the brain, Chiari malformation, and cranial aneurysm. There also is an online brain quiz. The Physician Resources section includes referral guidelines for conditions such as carpal tunnel syndrome as well as transcripts of chats on shaken baby syndrome, concussion and sports-related injuries, and low back pain. Neurosurgery On Call also hosts the online, peer-reviewed journal *Neurosurgical Focus*.

Orthopedic Surgery

American Academy of Orthopaedic Surgeons (http://www.aaos.org)

Special features on this Web page include a search function, what's new, annual meeting information, a product catalog, and the orthopedic yellow pages. A free benefit to members in the American Academy of Orthopaedic Surgeons is the creation of a personalized physician Web page for private practice. A photograph, educational background, and a map for United States and Canadian addresses may be included. An "Outlines and Guidelines" section includes six symptom-based clinical guidelines, including low back, knee, shoulder, hip, and wrist pain.

American Association of Orthopaedic Foot and Ankle Surgeons (http://www.footdocs.org)

This Web page details membership in the society, lists the state representatives for the organization, and has a members-only section called the "Coding Corner." In the Coding Corner, members may post a query to

Dr. Tye Ouzounian, an expert on coding and reimbursement for orthopedic procedures. The reply is sent via return e-mail. Information on how to join the society as well as a list of current board members are included. A password-protected bulletin board for members of the association is an opportunity to post questions and announcements regarding regional issues in foot and ankle care. An ambassador program promotes orthopedic surgeons as the premier providers of care for the foot and includes a study finding podiatric are 43% more expensive than orthopedic care.

American College of Sports Medicine (http://www.acsm.org)

The American College of Sports Medicine (ACSM) Web page contains a media room with news releases, quotes, "In the News," and history sections (Figure 12.9). The meeting and continuing education sections list the upcoming scientific meeting with highlights and a summary of each meeting stated. A member services center explains the benefits of becoming an ACSM member, describes each of the membership categories available, and allows application for new or renewal membership. Links to online journals, brochures, video and audio resources, and reference guides are available.

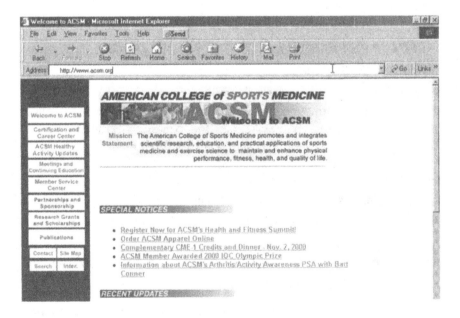

FIGURE 12.9. The Web page for the American College of Sports Medicine. (Reprinted with permission from David Brewer.)

Otolaryngologic Surgery

Acoustic Neuroma Association (http://anausa.org)

The Acoustic Neuroma Association was founded in 1981. It furnishes information on patient rehabilitation, promotes research, educates the public regarding the disease, and, most importantly, lists symptoms suggestive of acoustic neuroma. This Web page answers frequently asked questions such as "What is an acoustic neuroma?"; "What is your acoustic nerve and what does it do?"; "What causes acoustic neuromas?"; and others. A review of the treatment options for the disease, including microsurgical removal and stereotactic radiosurgery, are discussed. A section on life after acoustic neuroma surgery details the immediate postoperative care, the complications of spinal leak and hearing loss, and tinnitus as well as facial weakness or paralysis and eye problems. This Web page includes a glossary of terms and is an excellent reference for patients diagnosed with acoustic neuroma.

American Academy of Otolaryngology Surgery (http://www.entnet.org)

The American Academy of Otolaryngology Surgery is the world's largest group of physicians who routinely treat disorders of the ear, nose and throat, and head and neck. Among items on the academy's Web page, which is user friendly for patients and doctors alike, is the proper phonetic spelling of the specialty. Patients can click on the "Patient Info" section and learn "What Is an Otolaryngologist," take a fact and fiction quiz, and even find a specialist in their area. Specific diagnoses and symptoms are covered in well-written essays about topics such as "Ears, Altitude, and Flying," "Cochlear Implants," and "Buying a Hearing Aid." Under the Education section is an online medical student syllabus, a listing of continuing medical education programs and products, and a calendar of meetings. A thorough links section makes this Web site one of the very first to visit in this specialty.

American Board of Otolaryngology (http://www.aboto.org)

The American Board of Otolaryngology strives to progressively raise the quality of patient care in head and neck surgery. On this Web page, (Figure 12.10) one may find Microsoft Word or Corel WordPerfect documents containing important dates of concern to the practicing otolaryngologic surgeon. The Otolaryngology Training Examination (OTE) is covered in

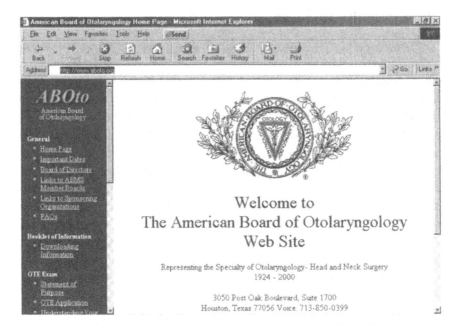

FIGURE 12.10. The American Board of Otolaryngology Web site. (Reprinted with permission from Caryn Wilson.)

detail on this Web page. A statement of purpose, candid guidelines, and a section entitled "Understanding Your Score Report" are included. Applications for the OTE are available on the Web page, and these also are in Word or WordPerfect format. Information concerning the cumulative log of surgical procedures performed in training is included. Finally, a map and directions to the board's Houston office are available.

American Neurotology Society (http://itsa.ucsf.edu/~ajo/ANS/ANS.html)

The purpose of the American Neurotology Society is "to exchange and disseminate information about the sensory-neural systems of audition and equilibrium." A history is included on this succinct Web page. Numerous policy statements of the society are listed online, such as the role that an otolaryngologist who limits practice to otology and neurotology should play in covering general head and neck surgery in the emergency room. There are three scholarships. The current and past officers as well as the William F. House Lectureship of the society are available on the Web page. A list of members and information on how to apply for membership also are included. A section for upcoming meetings is presented, and abstracts may be submitted electronically from this page. A newsletter keeps surgeons up to date on the society's activities.

American Rhinologic Society (http://www.american-rhinologic.org)

The American Rhinologic Society promotes excellence in clinical and basic science education in the field of rhinology and sinusology. Visitors to this site will find informative topics such as "An Introduction to Nasal Endoscopy," "New Surgical Techniques," and "Brief Overview of Sinus and Nasal Anatomy." These are all written essays that contain diagrams and photographs, all of which are geared to the level of a patient or nurse. Interested head and neck surgeons can find travel information for the upcoming meeting, review abstracts of previous meetings, or submit an abstract online. Three research grants, each valued at $10,000, are available from the society and are described on this Web page.

H.E.A.R. (Hearing Education and Awareness for Rockers) (http://www.hearnet.com)

This is a nonprofit organization with the goal of educating people on the dangers of repeated exposure to excessive noise levels, which as this Web page states, can lead to permanent, and sometimes debilitating, hearing loss and tinnitus. This Web page includes links to ear mold and monitor manufacturers as well as a list of HEARNET affiliate hearing professionals.

Support for People with Oral and Head and Neck Cancer (http://www.spohnc.org)

This Web page, produced by Support for People with Oral and Head and Neck Cancer, Inc., describes helpful hints for patients with malignant tumors of the head and neck. Many original articles are available here covering information about research studies, smoking, humor, the immune system, money matters, and oral care. An online membership and a listing of products to help improve the quality of life of people with oral and head and neck cancer are available. These include products to help relieve dry mouth, stimulate salivary flow, soothe the oral mucosa and lips, and oral hygiene products and preparations to protect the teeth. While none of these products is officially endorsed by the society, there are helpful links to these products that can help patients with oral cancers.

Wide Smiles, Cleft Lip, and Palate Resource (http://www.widesmiles.org)

Wide Smiles, founded in 1991, is a patient resource for parents with children born with cleft lips and/or palates. This Web page includes information on surgery to correct these disorders. Included here are important questions to ask your doctor, how to choose your surgeon, and the "Internet Guide to HMOs." Sections on insurance issues and Pierre Robin syndrome are included. Before and after photographs of children who have undergone reconstructive surgery to correct cleft lips and palates are displayed. The "Terms and Definitions" section is a good place to direct patients for information about the basic pathophysiology of these congenital defects.

Pediatric Surgery

American Pediatric Surgical Association (http://www.easpa.org)

The Web page for the American Pediatric Surgery Association contains a calendar of upcoming meetings that includes links to the hotels where the meetings are held. A directory of members lists phone and fax numbers as well as e-mail addresses in many cases. PEDSURG-L is a listserver housed online at the Robert Wood Johnson Medical School. Through it, actual patient problems on subjects such as "atresia with apple peel deformity" are discussed by pediatric surgeons. A links section is available.

Canadian Association of Pediatric Surgeons (http://www.caps.ca)

The Canadian Association of Pediatric Surgeons Web page outlines training objectives for medical students, surgery residents, pediatric residents, and pediatric surgery fellows. Listed for medical students as essential to diagnose are appendicitis, testicular torsion, and 26 other conditions. Similar goals for higher training are noted. Guidelines for referral to a pediatric surgeon for common childhood ailments, such as constipation, are available. Features that differentiate Hirschprung's disease from functional constipation are included in the later example. A short bowel syndrome study is under way, and the protocol and consent forms are available at this Web page.

Pediatric Burns (*http://www.pediatricburns.com*)

The home page for University Children's Hospital, Zurich, Switzerland, is one of the few sites in this highly specialized field. Although much of the information is locally based, a links section includes topics such as burn centers, literature, prevention, and support groups.

World of Pediatric Surgery (*http://www.pediatricsurgery.net*)

Visitors to the World of Pediatric Surgery first are greeted by an online poll inquiring about the visitors' opinions on controversial subjects in the field of pediatric surgery. After answering, the responses of all others polled are displayed to see how opinions compare. A Web page rich in information about laparoscopic pediatric surgery, this site includes original abstracts on topics such as immunologic benefits of laparoscopic surgery and tolerance to surgery of infants.

Plastic and Reconstructive Surgery

American Academy of Facial Plastic and Reconstructive Surgery (*http://www.facial-plastic-surgery.org*)

This organization, founded in 1964, has 2,600 members and is the world's largest association of specialists in facial plastic and reconstructive surgery. On this Web page, one can find a surgeon by zip code, last name, city, or country. The online bookstore includes *The Face Book*, which may be ordered directly from the Web page. Online patient brochures include pictures and discussions about topics such as blepharoplasty, scar revision, forehead lifts, hair replacement, and rhinoplasty. A media kit includes an extensive glossary of terms, common procedures on teenagers, cosmetic concerns and their corresponding dietary remedies, and a host of other topics.

American Society for Aesthetic Plastic Surgery (*http://surgery.org*)

The American Society for Aesthetic Plastic Surgery (ASAPS) is a not-for-profit organization that strives to educate and inform patients who are planning cosmetic plastic surgery. A "Find a Surgeon" section provides a geographic listing of ASAPS members. Under the "Procedures" section is an introduction to the various surgical procedures offered by cosmetic and plastic surgeons. A media center includes frequently updated topics of interest to the practicing plastic surgeon in a press release format. A patient gallery shows before and after pictures of real patients and provides the names of the plastic surgeons who performed those procedures. Specific procedures discussed include forehead lift, facelift, skin resurfacing, breast augmentation, lift and reduction, and abdominoplasty.

Lipoinfo (http://www.lipoinfo.com)

This site boasts that it is the most comprehensive liposuction information Web site on the entire Internet. The purpose of this site is to help individuals determine if they would benefit from liposuction and what type they might consider. It is intended for use by the general public and contains a glossary, tables, and extensive photos. It is divided into 42 sections, including the benefits of tumescent liposuction, ultrasonic liposuction, and sections on topics such as "Can fat grow back?" The benefits of having the procedure performed in the hospital rather than in an office also are covered. A section on questions to ask your surgeon includes nine important items to ask a surgeon prior to having this procedure. It includes "Is the doctor fully covered by malpractice for liposuction procedures?" This is frequently updated by Dr. Paul Weber, the author of the information sections of the Web page.

Plastic Surgery Information Services (http://www.plasticsurgery.org)

This is the Web page for the American Society of Plastic Surgeons and Plastic Surgery Educational Foundation (Figure 12.11). It contains statistics on a variety of topics in plastic surgery, including cosmetic and reconstructive procedure trends, gender and age distribution, average surgeon fees, and breast surgery statistics. The top five cosmetic procedures from 1992 to 1998 are listed, and they include liposuction, breast augmentation, eyelid surgery, facelift, and chemical peel. Each of the more popular procedures is listed in an illustrated patient information section. Topics include type of anesthesia, preparing for surgery, risks of surgery, and best candidates for a particular procedure. A key word search allows individual topics to be rapidly identified within the large Web page. News releases aimed at patients and physician papers focusing on health care professionals round out this extensive Web page.

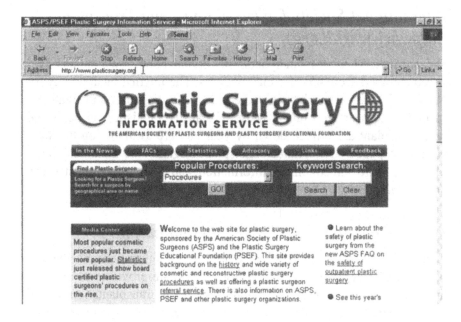

FIGURE 12.11. The Plastic Surgery Information Service. (Reprinted with permission from Nancy E. Ryan.)

Transplant Surgery

American Society of Transplantation (http://www.astp.org)

The American Society of Transplantation is an organization composed of 1,300 transplant surgeons, supporting doctors, and scientists who are dedicated to bettering the field of transplantation surgery. On the society's Web page, one may find the bylaws, mission, and membership of the organization. Upcoming meetings are listed, and the presidential address and abstracts from prior meetings are posted. A job bank is included and is frequently updated. A public policy section discusses the current controversial issues in transplantation and their status in the legislature.

International Society for Heart and Lung Transplant (http://www.ishlt.org)

Created in 1981 with 15 members, this organization now contains over 2,200 members from 45 different countries. The International Society for Heart and Lung Transplant is dedicated to the diagnosis and treatment of end-stage heart and lung disease. Exhaustive statistics on heart and lung transplant are broken down by year and are available on the society's Web page under "Annual Transplant Registry." A membership application, board and committee information, and heart failure registry also are available.

Organ Donation (http://www.organdonor.gov)

Created by Health Resources and Services Administration and the Department of Health and Human Services, this site provides information and resources on organ donation and issues about transplantation. Listed are organizations specializing in organ procurement, transplant networks, and government agencies. A common pop-culture myth about the man in the bathtub who wakes up and finds his kidneys have been harvested is dispelled.

Transplant Awareness, Inc. (http://www.transplantawareness.org)

This nonprofit corporation was founded and is operated by volunteers who have successfully undergone organ transplants. This group sells T-shirts ("Recycle yourself: be an organ and tissue donator"), books, pens, and stickers online. All proceeds from merchandise sales go to increasing organ and tissue transplantation awareness.

Transplant Patient Partnering (http://www.tppp.net)

The Transplant Patient Partnership Web page, which is a good resource for patients who have undergone or plan to undergo renal transplantation, is split into two main sections: "New Horizons: Pretransplant Preparation" and "New Beginnings: After Transplant Answers." Each is in a frequently asked questions format. Issues such as posttransplant diet and exercise are covered succinctly but thoroughly. A guide to sexual concerns after kidney transplants is included, as are discussions on finances, organ rejection, and the waiting list.

Transweb (http://www.transweb.org)

This busy Web site celebrated its fifth anniversary in 2000, making it one of the oldest Web pages about transplant surgery (Figure 12.12). Visitors may read in-depth answers to questions such as how many people in the United States are awaiting organ transplants (67,500) and whether kidneys may be sold (no). Donors and patients who died awaiting transplantation are memorialized with individual Web pages, many of which are quite touching. The site boasts that it contains over 10,000 items concerning all aspects of organ transplantation. A listing of centers is available and comprehensive.

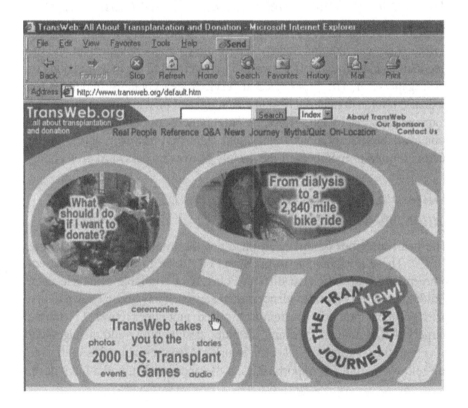

FIGURE 12.12. Transweb. (Reprinted with permission from Eleanor G. Jones.)

Trauma Surgery

American Association for the Surgery of Trauma (http://www.aast.org)

This site was created to promote the exchange of scientific information dealing with all aspects of the care of a trauma patient. Under the trauma resources section are links to other Web pages about trauma, guidelines for grading of specific organ injuries (e.g., liver and spleen), and Glasgow Coma Score outlines. A trauma prevention section contains an injury prevention guide, abstracts, and legislative alerts.

American Trauma Society (http://www.amtrauma.org)

An elaborate calendar of events for traumatologists highlights the Web page for the American Trauma Society. The society's mission statement and officers are included, as is the contact information for 22 state divisions of the organization. The programs and services area contains guidelines for pediatric trauma, a material resource catalog, and information about trauma courses sponsored by the society. An employment opportunities section lists jobs available for surgeons, nurses, and registrars; however, access to the area is limited to members of the society by way of password protection.

Eastern Association for the Surgery of Trauma (http://www.east.org)

The heart and soul of this Web page are the trauma guidelines (Figure 12.13). These are available in plain text or Adobe format. Levels of recommendation are based on different classes of available scientific data. Guidelines based on this evidence-based approach have been shown to improve clinical practice. Current completed guidelines cover 11 trauma surgery topics such as screening for blunt cardiac injury and management of penetrating intraperitoneal colon injuries. Also present on this Web page are fellowship and job opportunities, a membership list, and a links page.

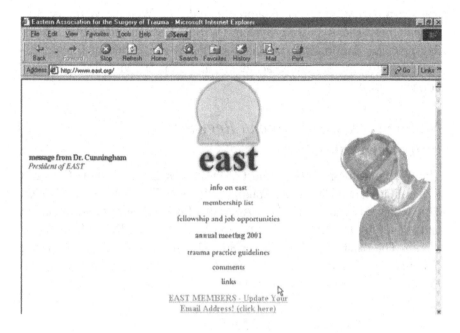

FIGURE 12.13. The Web page for Eastern Association for the Surgery of Trauma.

Emergency War Surgery
(http://www.vnh.org/EWSurg/EWSTOC.html)

Located with the Virtual Naval Hospital is the handbook for emergency war surgery. Edited by Drs. Thomas E. Bowen and Ronald Bellamy, this large document-turned–Web page covers topics such as mass injuries in thermonuclear war and wound profiles from an M-16 weapon. This site is a refreshingly simple look at surgery performed the military way. What is found online is an intriguing mix of illustrated surgical techniques, modern trauma care, and American history.

National Center for Injury Prevention and Control
(http://www.cdc.gov/ncipc/ncipchm.htm)

The National Center for Injury Prevention and Control has a goal of reducing morbidity, mortality, and costs associated with physical injuries. This Web page is a part of the vast site for the Centers for Disease Control (**http://www.cdc.gov**). Features include the Web-based Injury Statistics Query and Reporting System (WISQARS), an interactive system that provides data on injury-related mortality. Prevention of suicide, bicycle injuries, motor vehicle accidents, and domestic violence is a major point of interest.

National Pediatric Trauma Registry (http://www.nptr.org)

This Web page represents a project of the Research and Training Center in Rehabilitation and Childhood Trauma at the New England Medical Center. This registry is endorsed by the American Pediatric Surgical Association and funded by the National Institute on Disability and Rehabilitation Research. The database contains over 80,000 cases, and the 85 participating trauma centers contribute an additional 8,000 to 9,000 cases each year. Online submission or viewing the database is not available at present.

Society of Critical Care Medicine (http://www.sccm.org)

The Society of Critical Care Medicine is a nonprofit international organization with a mission to attain the highest quality of care for the critically ill patient. An ICU registry is available but is password protected. Employment opportunities and fellowship listings are present. Educational meeting schedules and critical care links are included. An easy-to-complete online application is available for those who want to join the society.

Trauma.org (http://www.trauma.org)

The trauma bank at this Web site contains a wealth of information about many subjects dealing with trauma. Each topic, such as injury prevention or vascular trauma, is covered with a featured article, mailing list discussions, Internet resources, and case presentations. The result is a broad base of clinical strategies and current opinion about a variety of subjects related to trauma. An image bank contains clinical and radiologic photographs of injuries that, in many cases, are quite illustrative.

Vascular Surgery

European Society for Vascular Surgery (http://www.esvs.org)

This organization, which was founded in May 1987, is one of the oldest vascular surgery Web pages, having been online since October 30, 1995. A world calendar of events of interest to the vascular surgeon is present. In addition, an elaborate list of links of vascular surgery Web sites is available. "Who's Who in Vascular Surgery" is a section that includes individual physician profiles from some of the leading vascular surgeons in the world. A comprehensive list of important vascular and endovascular trials is included and contains links to respective Web pages.

Journal of Vascular Surgery (http://www.mosby.com/jvs)

The Web page for the *Journal of Vascular Surgery*, sponsored in part by W.L. Gore & Associates, includes full text articles and abstracts from current issues of the *Journal of Vascular Surgery* as well as an archive that includes every issue since 1990. To obtain abstracts, no passwords are needed. However, to obtain the full-text online journal article, a subscription to the actual *Journal of Vascular Surgery* is necessary. Alternatively, the full-text articles may be viewed online by purchasing pay-for-view access for $25 each. This allows access to the article for 24 hours, at which time it is encouraged that the article be printed for future use at no additional cost. There is a search function for previous journal articles. The ability to order a subscription, reprints, and online access is available from this Web page.

Thrombosite (http://www.thrombosite.com)

This is the thrombolytic professional forum and resource center (Figure 12.14). This Web page includes research news, an online forum, case studies, and a list of links specific to coagulation disorders. A "Thromboglossary" contains definitions of terms related to the pathophysiology, pharmacology, and clinical aspects of thrombosis, thrombotic disorders, and hemostasis. An overview of the pathophysiology of heparin-associated thrombocytopenia is well written. Case studies include a brief history and a question and answer format. The drug information section includes links to the respective **http://www.pharminfo.com** location.

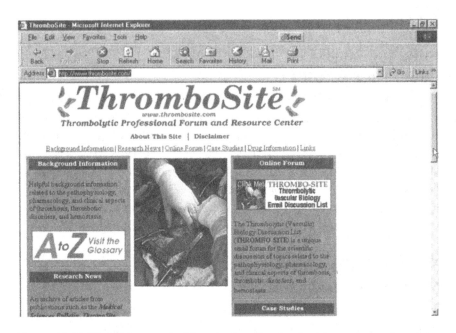

FIGURE 12.14. The Web page for Thrombosite. (Reprinted with permission from John Mack, VirSci Corporation.)

Vascular Surgery Societies Homepage (http://www.vascsurg.org)

Included on the Vascular Surgery Societies Homepage is the LifeLine Foundation, established in 1987 to promote and fund vascular surgery research among emerging young scientists. Information on how to apply to the LifeLine Foundation or for one of its annual awards is available. A case of the month illustrating unusual or challenging clinical problems is available. This site does, however, require a user identification and password from the society. A physician database, linked to Medline, and the *Journal of Vascular Surgery* are included. A frequently asked questions section answers queries such as "Who are vascular surgeons?"; "What kinds of problems do vascular surgeons treat?"; "What is an aneurysm?"; "What is a stroke?"; and "What causes varicose veins?"

General Surgery Products

Apligraf (http://www.apligraf.com)

Apligraf is a bioengineered wound care product made by Novartis Pharmaceuticals Corporation. It is a bilayered viable skin construct containing separate epidermal and dermal layers. The epidermal layer is formed by human keratinocytes, and the dermal layer contains human fibroblasts in a bovine type 1 collagen lattice. Apligraf helps achieve faster wound coverage and healing in data presented by Novartis.

Bard Perfix Plug (http://www.perfixplug.com)

Bard introduced this hernia repair system in 1993. It consists of two pieces of polypropylene mesh, one flat sheet and one that is molded into a tapered plug. Advocates of the "plug and patch" technique list decreased pain, fewer recurrences, and a shorter operative time as the main benefits. On the Web page is a free video offer, an online training session, frequently asked questions, a reference library, and a surgeons' resources area.

Composix (http://www.davol.com/composix.htm)

From the makers of the PerFix plug and patch system, this product is a hybrid form of mesh designed specifically for ventral hernia repair. One side of the mesh is polytetrafluoroethylene (PTFE) while the other side is polypropylene. The PTFE side faces the bowel and is said to prevent the adherence, and possible fistula formation, to the polypropylene. The polypropylene promotes ingrowth and adherence to the surrounding strength layers of the closure.

Cook (http://www.grii.com)

Cook group companies have been manufacturing quality surgical products since 1963. A history of the company and its innovators, including Sven-Ivan Seldinger, is presented. Each of Cook's individual companies, such as Cook Biotech Incorporated (**http://www.cookgroup.com/cook_biotech**), Cook Surgical (**http://www.cooksurgical.com**), and Wilson-Cook Medical (**http://www.wilsoncook.com**), are profiled and easily reached on the Web via links.

Ethicon (http://www.ethiconinc.com)

Here visitors will find information on a variety of surgical products made by Ethicon. An example is Panacryl, a braided synthetic absorbable suture. Panacryl has excellent retention of tensile strength without a permanent foreign body and associated reaction. The topical skin adhesive Dermabound is also described on this page. Information aimed at physicians and patients is presented separately. The package insert, advantages, instructions, and press releases are contained in the information for physicians. A separate Web page describes the Ethicon mesh hernia systems (**http://www.herniasolutions.com**).

Genzyme Surgical Products (http://www.genzyme.com)

Surgical products made by Genzyme include Seprafilm, Sepramesh, and a number of laparoscopic instruments. Each is described in detail at this Web page. Seprafilm is an innovative product that is designed to decrease postoperative adhesions. It acts as a barrier between surfaces of tissues that are prone to scar. The temporary shield helps to prevent adhesions because it keeps tissue surfaces separated during early wound healing, when adhesions are more prone to form.

Gore Medical (http://www.gore.com/medical/index.html)

This extensive Web page details the products made by Gore. The site is broken down anatomically. Under "legs," for example, are the vascular, casting, and orthopedic products. The endovascular and stretch grafts are described in the vascular section. Under "torso," the mesh used in ventral hernia repairs is detailed. The gynecologic, cardiothoracic, and bariatric surgical products that Gore produces also are discussed.

Harmonic Scalpel (http://www.harmonicscalpel.com)

An influential device introduced in 1993, the harmonic scalpel is used to divide tissues while securing hemostasis. This Web page describes the instrument, which is manufactured by Johnson & Johnson. Benefits of a harmonic scalpel include less thermal damage, minimal smoke, and no electrical current, which has its own inherent risks. This novel device is now commonly used in open and laparoscopic cholecystectomy, fundoplication, and colon resection.

Impra (*http://www.bardimpra.com*)

This page describes the products for vascular surgery made by Impra, a division of C. R. Bard, Inc. Impra designs vascular and endovascular grafts, knitted and woven polyester grafts, patches, fabrics, pledgets, carotid shunts, and vascular probes. Included online is a conference schedule of interest to vascular surgeons. This includes regional, national, and international events. In addition to detailing each of their products online, this Web page also includes information on training sessions. These are performed at the Arizona Heart Institute and the University of Chicago. Current workshop topics include anastomotic techniques for surgical residents and a program for dialysis unit personnel designed to prolong the life of access grafts.

Karl Storz (*http://www.karlstorz.com*)

From the makers of quality endoscopy equipment, this Web page is quite extensive. A company history, career information, and the world divisions of Karl Storz are included. The vast array of endoscopic products are described, including 10 procedural brochures, 13 catalogs, and 12 issues of *Endoworld*. Each may be ordered by filling out a simple online form. The Karl Storz products are displayed on the Web page, along with sales information.

Moss Tubes (*http://www.mosstubesinc.com/main.html*)

The makers of combination gastrostomy and jejunostomy feeding tubes outline their various products on this Web site. These have a benefit to patients who require jejunal feeds and simultaneous gastric decompression. A company profile, case histories, and a request for additional information are available. In addition, descriptions of each of the six different combination tubes are presented, including order information.

Neoprobe (*http://www.neoprobe.com*)

Neoprobe manufactures devices used in sentinel lymph node technologies as well as other gamma ray-guided surgery. On this Web page, visitors can visit the clinical education center. This area contains a list of training centers, a schedule of course offerings in lymphatic mapping and sentinel node biopsy, and a bibliography of journal articles. Also available are corporate information, investor relations, and a description of the company's investigational products, such as the RIGS technique using radiolabeled, tumor-specific targeting agent.

Stryker Instruments (**http://www.inst.strykercorp.com**)

Stryker makes instruments commonly used in orthopedic and general surgical procedures. A company profile and employment opportunities are presented in addition to details about their surgical products. The Stryker Pain Pump has its own page, located at **http://www.pain-pump.com**. The pump uses sustained vacuum pressure to deliver a continuous analgesic infusion at controlled rates directly to the operative site. Additionally, products from the endoscopic division of Stryker are available at **http://www.strykerendo.com**.

Tissue Sealing.com (**http://www.tissuesealing.com**)

This Web page, sponsored by Baxter, provides information on fibrin tissue adhesives for surgical sealing and hemostasis. At present, the product known as Tisseel, is approved in the United States for hemostasis during surgeries involving cardiopulmonary bypass, when treating traumatic splenic injuries, and during colostomy closure. In other areas of the world, the product is approved for tissue gluing and support of wound healing.

13
Health-Related Internet Resources

General Medicine

Many of the Web sites listed in the previous chapter have general surgery or a surgical specialty as their focus. The Web pages highlighted here fall more into the category of general medicine, although many have a section or sections dedicated to surgery. These pages typically are the highly trafficked sites with commercial appeal.

General Medicine

American Red Cross (http://www.redcross.org)

The Web page for the American Red Cross describes the functions of this large organization. It includes sections dedicated to armed forces emergency services, biomedical services, disaster services, nursing, youth development, and volunteering. The site offers the ability to donate to the Red Cross by credit card or donate stock shares. A virtual museum displays the activities of the Red Cross in six separate eras that span from before 1900 to the year 2000.

Centers for Disease Control (http://www.cdc.gov/)

The Web page for the Centers for Disease Control (CDC) details the many functions of this national organization. Health Topics A–Z alphabetically lists many health concerns of the general population. An especially useful area of the page is the Travelers' Health section (Figure 13.1), which describes useful recommendations for travelers going to a variety of destinations. Thoroughly discussed are geographic specific health threats, suggested immunizations, what not to eat or drink, and what you need to bring to stay healthy. Also, new products, such as Malarone (a fixed combination of atovaquone and proguanil hydrochloride), are described. Malarone is a new antimalarial drug approved for both treatment and prophylaxis of malaria.

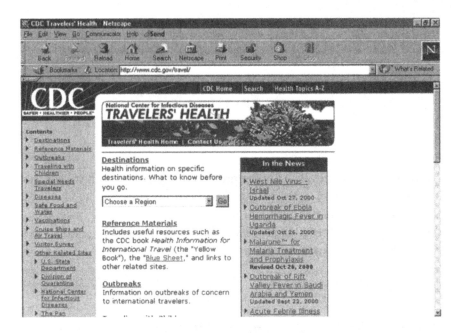

FIGURE 13.1. The Web page for the Centers for Disease Control Travelers' Health. (Reprinted with permission from CDC/Traveler's Health.)

Clinical Trials (*http://clinical trials.gov*)

A service of the National Institutes of Health through the National Library of Medicine, this Web page is aimed at the general public. It gives up-to-date information about ongoing clinical trials. Visitors may type in a disease or condition, and this site will search the Web and list all known ongoing clinical trials about the subject. In addition, a section entitled "Understanding Clinical Trials" alerts patients to the nature of trials and answers questions such as "What is a clinical trial?"; "Why should I volunteer for a trial?"; and "What questions should I ask?"

Dr. Koop (*http://www.drkoop.com*)

Founded by the former surgeon general, Dr. C. Everett Koop, this site advertises that "the best prescription is knowledge." Headlines, health policies, and recalls highlight the Health News portion of the page. Health Tools online include calculators for diabetes risk, visual acuity, sleep index, ideal body weight, and bladder control.

Healtheon (http://www.healtheon.com)

Now known as **webMD (http://www.webmd.com/)**
Under the consumer heading, webMD presents "health news and medical information for the general public." A new area lists common diseases and offers general guidelines to care. News stories about health care also are featured. Access to the physician section requires membership. In the physician section, there is an online version of *Scientific American Medicine*, a daily news feature, and the ability to create free personal medical Web pages.

Healthgate (http://www.healthgate.com)

In the patient area, there are over 250 topics available for review. Surgical conditions, such as gallstones, Crohn's disease, and hemorrhoids, each have dedicated sections that explain the basics of the diagnosis and treatment of each disease. The professionals' corner contains Medline, CME courses, and a daily review of heath-related news stories from Reuters.

Medscape (http://www.medscape.com)

Free membership entitles you to, among other features, Medline searches and a personal Web page. The latter will display office locations with maps, special instructions to patients, contact information, credentials, and links. The Medscape version of Medline offers highly customized searchers from 1960 to the present, is fast, and has an easy-to-use interface. Also available at Medscape are practice guidelines, conference summaries, and frequent advertisements.

Physicians Online (http://www.pol.net)

This site features discussion groups, Medline searches, drug interactions, new drugs under development, outlines in clinical medicine, clinical IQ, quizzes, and a medical bookstore. Membership, required to view most of the online material, is free and is available to U.S. physicians (M.D.s and D.O.s), physicians-in-training, and medical students.

PubMed (http://www.ncbi.nlm.nih.gov/entrez/query.fcgi?db=PubMed)

PubMed is the National Library of Medicine's search service that provides access to over 10 million citations in MEDLINE, PreMEDLINE, and other similar databases. Alongside the searches are links to participating online journals, where available. The search function is quick, free, and may be customized. No passwords or memberships are needed to use PubMed.

14
Nonmedical Web Pages

Sports
News
Music
Cinema
Travel
Maps and Directions
Stock Market and Investing
All-In-One

While many of us often do not admit it, there is life outside of surgery. In addition to the numerous medical and surgical applications already discussed, there are many entertaining and personal uses of the Internet. Using the World Wide Web is a great way to find sports scores, make vacation plans, buy or sell goods, find music, or just pass some idle time "surfing."

Sports

For the sports enthusiast, the Internet offers scoreboards, behind-the-scenes stories, and in many cases, live video or audio broadcasts. Fantasy sports, where participants act as owners, managers, and coaches of selected professional athletes, are taken to a new level by the Web.

Sports fans will want to start by visiting *Sports Illustrated*'s Web page (**http://www.cnnsi.com**), made in partnership with Cable News Network (CNN). In addition to the comprehensive scoreboards and league standings in all major sports, there is an area dedicated to audio and video clips entitled "multimedia central." Here, viewers may pick from a variety of interviews and game highlights and play them online using the Real Audio player (downloaded for free at **http://www.realaudio.com**).

News

The Web page for the Cable News Network (CNN) is an excellent place to get caught up with the day's newsworthy events. Located at **http://www.cnn.com**, it contains all the breaking stories worldwide. Spinoff Web sites include CNN Europe (**http://europe.cnn.com**), CNN financial network (**http://cnnfn.cnn.com**), and CNN for students (**http://fyi.cnn.com/fyi**). Outside CNN, scaled-down news Web pages may be found at Netscape (**http://home.netscape.com**), The Wire (**http://wire.ap.org**), and Lycos (**www.lycos.com/news**).

Music

One of the most popular sites in the entire World Wide Web is the Web page for Music Television (**http://www.mtv.com**). Visitors here are greeted with headlines and stories about popular music and the bands that create it; tour schedules for many groups; and the ability to view selected music video clips. The Web page for sister station VH-1 (**http://www.vh1.com**) is similarly enjoyable and contains more mainstream music with less cutting edge and hard-rock groups.

The Internet also has spawned an entirely new way of buying, storing, and playing music called MP3. MP3 stands for Moving Picture Expert Group-1, Audio Layer-3. It is a format for compressing a sound sequence into a very small file. MP3s have superior sound quality and take up relatively small amounts of computer memory. Certain MP3 files may be legally downloaded from reputable Web pages, such as **http://www.mp3.com**. Other MP3s (usually popular, copyrighted material) are considered contraband, but can still be found on some illegal Web pages. MP3s may be played over the computer's speakers using special software, which is generally free and often preinstalled on newer computers. Portable MP3 players are becoming popular; they can interface with the computer and transfer songs from the PC to the portable MP3 player.

Cinema

The World Wide Web offers many opportunities for moviegoers. Renting VHS and DVD titles is as easy as visiting NetFlix (**http://www.netflix.com**) or Rentvideosonthenet.com (**http://rentvideosonthenet.com/dvd**). Purchasing the movies is similarly easy. There is a large selection of titles available at Amazon (**http:www.amazon.com**) or CD-Now (**http://www.cdnow.com**). Movie buffs can learn much more about individual movies by visiting the Internet Movie Database (**http://www. imdb.com**) (Figure 14.1). Public ratings, goofs, trivia, memorable quotes, alternate endings, and much more are available for nearly every movie ever created.

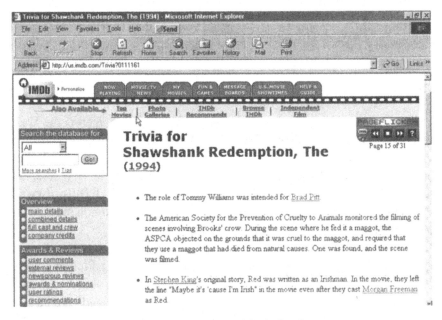

FIGURE 14.1. The Internet Movie Database.

Travel

Whether for work or leisure, the Internet markedly improves and simplifies travel planning. A visit to a digital travel agency will allow you to compare airfares, get tips on obtaining low fares, check frequent flyer mileage, and even select a seat assignment. Yahoo! Travel (**http:// travel.yahoo.com**), Lycos Travel (**http://travel.lycos.com**), Travelocity (**http://www.tavelocity.com**), and Concierge.com (**http://www.concierge. com**) are examples of these comprehensive travel sites. After booking a flight, visitors to these Web pages can reserve hotel rooms, find rental cars, and read reviews about destinations. Discounted airfare is available at flycheap (**www.flycheap.com**), lastminutetravel.com (**www.lastmin-utetravel.com**), and lowestfare.com (**www.lowestfare.com**).

Maps and Directions

Just as search engines assist in navigation of the World Wide Web, there are a few Web pages that can help you navigate the physical world. These include Yahoo Maps (**http://maps.yahoo.com**), Alta Vista Maps (**http:// tools.altavista.com/s?spage=t/map.htm**), and MapQuest (**http://www. mapquest.com**). Simply type in starting and destination points, and these Web pages will "connect the dots" and give detailed directions for travel from start to finish. Recently, a live traffic section has been added to the Map Quest site that includes a report on automobile accidents and a traffic cam for selected cities.

Stock Market and Investing

The online Stock Market, more than any other subject, has been a catalyst for surgeons to learn computing. The rapidity of trading online, coupled with convenience and markedly discounted commissions, has spawned a new form of investor, the day trader. There are a number of Web sites that bring the ability to buy and sell stocks, options, mutual funds, and bonds to your personal computer (Table 14.1). Other pages include financial planning, stock tips, statistics, and stories. The Motley Fool (**http://www.fool.com**), consistently ranked among the best investment Web pages, is an excellent place to start. This page details the rule breakers and rule makers that have made its creators (David and Tom Gardner) famous. *The Wall Street Journal* (**http://www.wsj.com**), CNNfn (**http://cnnfn.cnn.com**), and *Money Magazine* online (**http://www.money. com**) are laden with financial information.

TABLE 14.1. Online stock brokers.

Company	Commission per trade	Minimum balance	Realtime quotes	Web URL
Ameritrade	$8.00	$2,000	Free	**http://www.ameritrade.com**
E-trade	$14.95 to $19.95	$1,000	Free	**http://www.etrade.com**
Schwab	$14.95 to $29.95	$5,000	Free	**http://www.schwab.com**
Datek	$9.99	None	Free	**http://www.datek.com**
TD Waterhouse	$12.00 to $15.00	$1,000	Free	**http://www.waterhouse.com**

All-In-One

David Filo and Jerry Yang created Yahoo! to keep up with their personal Web interests. While Yahoo! has instead evolved into a search engine, the My Yahoo! feature does a good job fulfilling the duo's initial goal. A free service, My Yahoo! enables users to select certain of their fluctuating personal interests over which they would like to keep a close watch (Figure 14.2). Examples of items that may be included on a My Yahoo! page include headline news, local weather, television listings, stock portfolios with automatically updated balances, and best rates for mortgage, car loans, or airline travel. A dynamic calendar is available that allows appointments to be entered or viewed from any computer connected to the Internet. In addition, the calendar will interface with many personal digital assistants, such as Palm Pilots. Many rivals to the Yahoo! search engine have their own "my" pages. This includes My Lycos (**http://www.lycos.com**), My Alta Vista (**http://www.altavista.com**), and My Excite (**http://www.excite.com**).

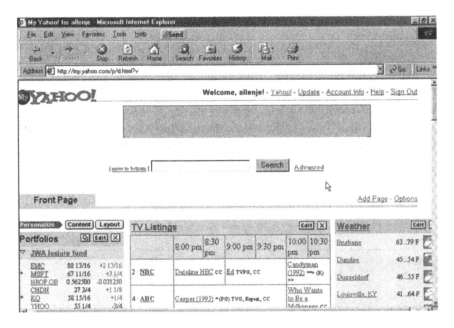

FIGURE 14.2. My Yahoo! Page for the author.

Appendix I
Web Pages for Departments of Surgery in the United States

Alabama
    University of Alabama Birmingham
      (**http://main.uab.edu/uasom/2/show.asp?durki=23194**)
    University of South Alabama
      (**http://www.usouthal.edu/ResidencyPrograms/surgery.html**)

Arizona
    University of Arizona (**http://www.surgery.arizona.edu**)

Arkansas
    University of Arkansas (**http://surgery.uams.edu**)

California
    Cedars-Sinai (**http://www.csmc.edu/gme/surgery/programs.htm**)
    University of California–Davis
      (**http://web.ucdmc.ucdavis.edu/surgery**)
    University of California–Irvine (**http://www.ucihs.uci.edu/surgery**)
    University of California–Los Angeles (**http://149.142.102.4**)
    University of California–San Diego (**http://www-surgery.ucsd.edu**)
    University of California–San Francisco (**http://www.surgery.ucsf.edu**)
    University of Southern California (**http://www.surgery.usc.edu**)
    Stanford University (**http://surgeons.stanford.edu**)

Colorado
    University of Colorado (**http://www.uchsc.edu/sm/surgery**)

Connecticut
    Yale University (**http://yalesurgery.med.yale.edu**)

Florida
    Miami University
      (**http://www.um-jmh.org/guide/guide.asp?dept=Surgery**)
    University of Florida (**http://www.surgery.ufl.edu**)

University of South Florida
(**http://com1.med.usf.edu/SURGERY/division.html**)

Georgia
Emory University
(**http://www.emory.edu/WHSC/MED/SURGERY**)
Medical College of Georgia
(**http://www.mcg.edu/SOM/Surgery/Index.html**)

Hawaii
University of Hawaii
(**http://medworld.biomed.Hawaii.Edu/HRP/gensubro.html**)

Illinois
Fitch University (**http://www.finchcms.edu/Surgery/surgery.htm**)
Loyola University Chicago
(**http://www.meddean.luc.edu/ssom/depts/patcar/gensur.htm**)
Northwestern University
(**http://surgery.nwu.edu/content/index.html**)
Rush (**http://www.rush.edu/patients/surgery/index.html**)
Southern Illinois University (**http://www.siumed.edu/surgery**)
University of Chicago (**http://www-surgery.bsd.uchicago.edu**)
University of Illinois at Chicago
(**http://www.uic.edu/com/surgery/_private**)

Indiana
Indiana University (**http://scalpel.med.iupui.edu**)

Iowa
University of Iowa (**http://www.surgery.uiowa.edu**)

Kansas
University of Kansas–Witchita (**http://wichita.kumc.edu/surgery**)

Kentucky
University of Kentucky (**http://www.mc.uky.edu/surgery**)
University of Louisville (**http://www.louisvillesurgery.com**)

Louisiana
LSU
(**http://www.test.medschool.lsumc.edu/surgery/Academic/gen.htm**)
Tulane University (**http://www.tulane.edu/~surgery**)

Maryland

John Hopkins (**http://www.jhbmc.jhu.edu/Surgery/**)
University of Maryland
(**http://medschool.umaryland.edu/Departments/Surgery/**)

Massachusetts

Boston University (**http://www.bumc.bu.edu/Departments/
HomeMain.asp?DepartmentID=69**)
Harvard Medical School
(**http://www.hmcnet.harvard.edu/temp/surg.html**)
Tufts University
(**http://www.tufts.edu/med/dept/clinical/surg.html**)
University of Massachusetts (**http://www.umassmed.edusurgery**)

Michigan

Michigan State University
(**http://web2.chm.msu.edu/Surgery/CHM_ClinicalSurgery.htm**)
University of Michigan (**http://www.surgery.med.umich.edu**)
Wayne State University (**http://www.med.wayne.edu/surgery**)

Minnesota

Mayo Clinic (**http://www.mayo.edu/mgsm/rgs.htm**)
University of Minnesota (**http://www.surg.umn.edu**)

Mississippi

University of Mississippi (**http://surgery.umc.edu**)

Missouri

St. Louis University
(**http://medschool.slu.edu/departments/surgery**)
University of Missouri–Columbia
(**http://www.surgery.missouri.edu/care**)
University of Missouri–Kansas City
(**http://cctr.umkc.edu/dept/surgery/index.html**)
Washington University (**http://www.surgery.wustl.edu**)

Nebraska

Creighton University (**http://www.creighton.edu/Surgery**)

Nevada

University of Nevada (**http://www.unr.edu/med/surgerylk.html**)

New Hampshire
Dartmouth Medical Center (**http://www.hitchcock.org/pages/
DeptSurg/Surg_Pages/dos_main_page.htm**)

New Jersey
New Jersey Medical School (**http://www.umdnj.edu/njmsweb/surg**)
Robert Wood Johnson Medical School
(**http://rwjsurgery.umdnj.edu/default.html**)

New Mexico
University of New Mexico
(**http://hsc.unm.edu/som/acaddpts.html**)

New York
Albany Medical College
(**http://www.amc.edu/GME/surgery_residencies.htm**)
Albert Einstein University
(**http://www.aecom.yu.edu/home/surgery/surgery.htm**)
Columbia University (**http://www.columbiasurgery.org**)
Cornell University (**http://surgery.med.cornell.edu**)
Mt. Sinai Medical Center
(**http://www.mssm.edu/surgery/home-page.html**)
New York Medical College
(**http://www.nymc.edu/depthome/academic/surgery/surgery.htm**)
New York University (**http://www.med.nyu.edu**)
SUNY Buffalo (**http://wings.buffalo.edu/smbs/sur**)
SUNY Downstate (**http://www.hscbklyn.edu/Surgery/default.html**)
SUNY Stony Brook
(**http://www.uhmc.sunysb.edu/surgery/edu/general**)
SUNY Syracuse (**http://www.universityhospital.org/surgery**)

North Carolina
Duke University (**http://surgery.mc.duke.edu**)
East Carolina University (**http://www.surgery.ecu.edu**)
University of North Carolina (**http://www.med.unc.edu/cgi-bin/
partialIndex.pl/wrkunits/2depts/surgery**)
Wake Forrest (**http://isnet.is.wfu.edu/bgsm/surg-sci/gs/gs.html**)

North Dakota
University of North Dakota
(**http://www.med.und.nodak.edu/depts/surgery/clerk/home.htm**)

Ohio

Case Western
(**http://mediswww.meds.cwru.edu/som/surgaffils.html**)
Ohio State University (**http://www-surgery.med.ohio-state.edu**)
University of Cincinnati (**http://surgery.uc.edu**)
Wright State University
(**http://www.med.wright.edu/som/academic/surgery/division.htm**)

Oklahoma

University of Oklahoma (**http://w3.uokhsc.edu/surgery/**)

Pennsylvania

MCP Hahnemann
(**http://www.mcphu.edu/medschool/depts/surgery.html**)
Penn State Geisinger (**http://www.collmed.psu.edu/surg**)
Temple University (**http://blue.temple.edu/~tums/departments/
clinical/Surgery/Department.html**)
Thomas Jefferson University
(**http://jeffline.tju.edu/CWIS/DEPT/Surgery**)
University of Pennsylvania
(**http://health.upenn.edu/surgery/index.html**)
University of Pittsburgh (**http://www.surgery.upmc.edu**)

Rhode Island

Brown University
(**http://www.brown.edu/Departments/Surgery/pages/program.html**)

South Carolina

Medical University of South Carolina (**http://www.musc.edu/surgery**)
University of South Carolina
(**http://www.prmh.edu/residency/surgical.html**)

South Dakota

University of South Dakota (**http://med.usd.edu/surg**)

Tennessee

East Tennessee State (**http://www.etsu.edu/surgery**)
Meharry Medical College
(**http://www.mmc.edu/medschool/ClinicalSci/Surgery/Default.htm**)
University of Tennessee
(**http://www.utmem.edu/surgery/pub/residency.html**)
Vanderbilt University (**http://www.mc.vanderbilt.edu/surgery**)

Texas

Baylor University (**http://www.bcm.tmc.edu/surgery**)
Texas A&M University (**http://tamushsc.tamu.edu/SURG.html**)
Texas Tech University
(**http://www.ttuhsc.edu/pages/surgery/default.html**)
University of Texas–Galveston (**http://www.utmb.edu/surgery**)
University of Texas–Houston
(**http://utsurg.med.uth.tmc.edu/index.html**)
University of Texas–Southwestern
(**http://www.swmed.edu/home_pages/surgery**)

Utah

University of Utah (**http://www.med.utah.edu/surgery**)

Vermont

University of Vermont (**http://www.vtmednet.org/surgery**)

Virginia

Eastern Virginia Medical School
(**http://www.evms.edu/surgery/index.html**)
University of Virginia
(**http://hsc.virginia.edu/medicine/clinical/surgery**)
Virginia Commonwealth University (**http://www.surgery.vcu.edu**)

Washington

University of Washington (**http://depts. washington.edu/surgery**)

Washington, DC

George Washington University
(**http://www.gwumc.edu/edu/surgery/index.htm**)
Georgetown University
(**http://www.dml.georgetown.edu/schmed/depts/surgery.html**)
Howard University (**http://www.huhosp.org/surgery/default.htm**)

West Virginia

Marshall University (**http://meb.marshall.edu/medctr/surgery**)
West Virginia University (**http://www.hsc.wvu.edu/som/surgery**)

Wisconsin

Medical College of Wisconsin (**http://www.mcw.edu/surgery**)
University of Wisconsin (**http://www.surgery.wisc.edu**)

Appendix II
International Domain Suffixes and Common Top-Level Domains

International Domain Suffixes

A

Afghanistan	AF
Albania	AL
Algeria	DZ
American Samoa	AS
Andorra	AD
Angola	AO
Anguilla	AI
Antarctica	AQ
Antigua and Barbuda	AG
Argentina	AR
Armenia	AM
Aruba	AW
Australia	AU
Austria	AT
Azerbaijan	AZ

B

Bahamas	BS
Bahrain	BH
Bangladesh	BD
Barbados	BB
Belarus	BY
Belgium	BE
Belize	BZ
Benin	BJ
Bermuda	BM
Buhtan	BT
Bolivia	BO
Bosnia-Herzegovina	BA
Botswana	BW

Bouvet Island	BV
Brazil	BR
British Indian Ocean Territory	IO
Brunei Darussalam	BN
Bulgaria	BG
Burkina Faso	BF
Burundi	BI

C

Cambodia	KH
Cameroon	CM
Canada	CA
Cape Verde	CV
Cayman Islands	KY
Central African Republic	CF
Chad	TD
Chile	CL
China	CN
Christmas Island	CX
Cocos (Keeling) Islands	CC
Colombia	CO
Comoros	KM
Congo	CG
Cook Islands	CK
Costa Rica	CR
Croatia (Hrvatska)	HR
Cuba	CU
Cyprus	CY
Czech Republic	CZ
Czechoslovakia	CS

D

Democratic Republic of Congo	CD
Denmark	DK
Djibouti	DJ
Dominica	DM
Dominican Republic	DO

E

East Timor	TP
Ecuador	EC
Egypt	EG
El Salvador	SV
Equatorial Guinea	GQ
Estonia	EE
Ethiopia	ET

F

Falkland Islands (Malvinas)	FK
Faroe Islands	FO
Fiji	FJ
Finland	FI
France	FR
France (European Territory)	FX
French Guyana	GF
French Polynesia	PF
French Southern Territories	TF

G

Gabon	GA
Gambia	GM
Georgia	GE
Germany	DE
Ghana	GH
Gibraltar	GI
Greece	GR
Greenland	GL
Grenada	GD
Guadeloupe (French)	GP
Guam (U.S.)	GU
Guatemala	GT

Guinea	GN
Guinea-Bissau	GW
Guyana	GY

H

Haiti	HT
Heard and McDonald Islands	HM
Honduras	HN
Hong Kong	HK
Hungary	HU

I

Iceland	IS
India	IN
Indonesia	ID
Islamic Republic of Iran	IR
Iraq	IQ
Ireland	IE
Israel	IL
Italy	IT
Ivory Coast (Côte D'Ivoire)	CI

J

Jamaica	JM
Japan	JP
Jordan	JO

K

Kazakhstan	KZ
Kenya	KE
Kiribati	KI
Kuwait	KW
Kyrgyzstan	KG

L

Laos (People's Democratic Republic)	LA
Latvia	LV
Lebanon	LB
Lesotho	LS

Liberia	LR	Niger	NE
Libya (Libyan Arab	LY	Nigeria	NG
Jamahiriya)		Niue	NU
Liechtenstein	LI	Norfolk Island	NF
Lithuania	LT	North Korea	KP
Luxembourg	LU	Northern Mariana Islands	MP
		Norway	NO

M

Macau	MO
Macedonia (Former	
Yugoslav Republic of)	MK
Madagascar	MG
Malawi	MW
Malaysia	MY
Maldives	MV
Mali	ML
Malta	MT
Marshall Islands	MH
Martinque (French)	MQ
Mauritania	MR
Mauritius	MU
Mexico	MX
Micronesia	FM
Moldavia	MD
Monaco	MC
Mongolia	MN
Montserrat	MS
Morocco	MA
Mozambique	MZ
Myanmar	MM

N

Namibia	NA
Nauru	NR
Nepal	NP
Netherland Antilles	AN
Netherlands	NL
Neutral Zone	NT
New Caledonia (French)	NC
New Zealand	NZ
Nicaragua	NI

O

Oman	OM

P

Pakistan	PK
Palau	PW
Panama	PA
Papua New Guinea	PG
Paraguay	PY
Peru	PE
Philippines	PH
Pitcairn	PN
Poland	PL
Polynesia (French)	PF
Portugal	PT
Puerto Rico (U.S.)	PR

Q

Qatar	QA

R

Reunion (French)	RE
Romania	RO
Russian Federation	RU
Rwanda	RW

S

Saint Helena	SH
Saint Kitts Nevis Anguilla	KN
Saint Lucia	LC
Saint Pierre and Miquelon	PM
Saint Tome and Principe	ST

Saint Vincent and the Grenadines	VC	Trinidad and Tobago	TT
		Tunisia	TN
Samoa	WS	Turkey	TR
San Marino	SM	Turkmenistan	TM
Saudi Arabia	SA	Turks and CAicos Islands	TC
Senegal	SN	Tuvalu	TV
Seychelles	SC		
Sierra Leone	SL	**U**	
Singapore	SG	Uganda	UG
Slovak Republic (Slovakia)	SK	Ukraine	UA
Slovenia	SI	United Arab Emirates	AE
Solomon Islands	SB	United Kingdom	UK
Somalia	SO	United States of America	US
South Africa	ZA	United States Minor Outlying Islands	UM
South Korea	KR		
Soviet Union	SU	Uruguay	UY
Spain	ES	Uzbekistan	UZ
Sri Lanka	LK		
Sudan	SD	**V**	
Surinam	SR	Vanuatu	VU
Svalbard and Jan Mayen Islands	SJ	Vatican City State	VA
		Venezuela	VE
Swaziland	SZ	Vietnam	VN
Sweden	SE	Virgin Islands (British)	VG
Switzerland	CH	Virgin Islands (US)	VI
Syria (Syrian Arab Republic)	SY		
		W	
T		Wallis and Futuna Islands	WF
Taiwan	TW	Western Sahara	EH
Tajikistan	TJ	**Y**	
Tanzania	TZ	Yemen	YE
Thailand	TH	Yugoslavia	YU
Togo	TG		
Tokelau	TK	**Z**	
Tonga	TO	Zambia	ZM

Common Top-Level Domains

.com   Commercial
.edu   Educational
.gov   Government
.int   International
.mil   United States military
.net   Network infrastructure
.org   Nonprofit organization

Note: Recently, a second flight of top-level domains have been added and are available for public use. This includes .tv, .cc, and .ws. Interestingly, .tv is the international Domain Suffix for the country of Tuvalu. Through a financial arrangement with Tuvalu, .tv became a registrar for names in this domain. Tuvalu plans to use proceeds, estimated at over $4 million annually, to increase the quality of life for its population of approximately 10,000 citizens.

Glossary

Adobe   The company that makes Acrobat, a piece of software that displays documents in an easy to read and print format. Files that Acrobat reads have a ".pdf" extension.

Applet   A small program that works with Web pages to produce effects that are beyond the scope of standard HTML.

ARPA   Advanced Research Projects Agency. One of the organizations created by the Department of Defense to study new technologies.

ARPAnet   Advanced Research Projects Agency network. One of the precursors to the modern Internet.

Attachment   A file that is sent along with a piece of electronic mail. It may be a graphic, text, or sound file.

Bandwidth   Literally means a measure of the range of frequencies the signal occupies. In use, it is directly proportional to the amount of data transmitted or received per unit time (large bandwidth = more data).

Baud   Older nomenclature used to describe the amount of data transferred per second over a modem. Although not literally, it has been used synonymously with the newer measure of bps, or bits per second.

Bit   The smallest unit of data. A number in base 2 (0 or 1) occupies one bit.

Browser   Program that displays Web pages. Examples include Microsoft Internet Explorer and Netscape Navigator.

Byte   A unit of data. Eight bits make up one byte. A letter in the alphabet usually is one byte.

Cable modem	A connection to the Internet using a special device from a cable company that can send and receive data at nearly 1.5 Mbps.
CD-ROM	Compact disc–read only memory. A shiny disc that houses a large amount of computerized data. Identical in appearance to music compact discs.
Chat room	Specialized Web page that allows typed messages to be circulated among visitors, usually about a specific subject.
.com	commercial. The suffix for a commercial Web page.
Cookie	A piece of information that is sent from a Web server to your browser. The browser stores and remembers the cookie and then returns it to the server on later visits, as needed. Frequent uses of cookies include remembering passwords for log in to certain Web pages.
Crash	An event where the computer no longer properly responds. Often due to a virus. There are varying levels of computer crashes.
Cyberspace	A word coined by William Gibson in his novel *Neuromancer*. It is often used as a synonym to Internet, but really can pertain to information and resources made available by computer networks.
Domain name	Used synonymously with Web address and Uniform Resource Locator, this is the unique name that identifies a specific Web page.
Download	The transfer of material from a remote computer to a local, usually smaller, one.
DSL	Digital Subscriber Line. A method for rapid data transfer over conventional telephone lines.
DVD	Digital video disc (also digital versatile disc). These storage and playback discs can hold video, audio, and/or computer data.
E-commerce	Using the Internet to conduct business involving buying and/or selling.
E-mail	Electronic mail. The system of sending typed messages to another person using the Internet.

Encryption

The conversion of files into a form that cannot be easily recognized or interpreted without authorization.

Ethernet

A very fast system of data transfer based on a local area network.

FAQ

Frequently asked questions.

Floppy disk/drive

A temporary storage device for small amounts of data.

Freeware

Software that is offered at no cost. It can be freely distributed, but not sold or incorporated into other programs for sales.

FTP

File Transfer Protocol. This is one of the ways that individual files are exchanged between two or more remote users on the Internet.

GIF

One of the two main image formats that are displayed on Web pages (the g is pronounced like the j in jelly). Excellent for display of icons and on-line cartoons.

Gigabyte

A large amount of data, typically on the order of magnitude of the storage capacity of a hard drive. Literally, it is approximately 1,000 megabytes.

Hard drive

A nonremovable area of storage. It generally holds a large amount of data and is encased with the processor and other parts of the computer.

Hardware

Physical computer equipment such as a monitor, modem, printer, etc.

Hit

The number of visits to a Web page in a certain amount of time. Technically, each time someone views a Web page, it should be considered a hit. Like all attendance parameters, it is difficult to accurately measure and is easily inflated.

Home page

May be used interchangeably with Web page. Purists may point out that it means the opening or first page of a larger Web site.

HTML

HyperText Markup Language. The flexible, powerful programming language in which Web pages are written.

HTML editor	Program, similar to a word processor, that creates an HTML document. An HTML document also is known as a Web page.
HTPP	HyperText Transfer Protocol. The underlying system for information transfer on the Internet.
International domain suffix	A two-letter extension at the end of a Web page address that indicates the country of origin.
Internet	A system of interconnections of networks of computers allowing data transfer.
Internet telephony	The process of using the Internet to make telephone calls. This eliminates or markedly decreases long distance charges.
Intranet	A network inside a company, university, or similar large organization. It uses similar software as the Internet (browsers, e-mail, etc.) but is available only to members of the organization.
ISDN	Integrated Services Digital Network. A set of standards allowing digital transmission over copper wires making up telephone cable. Data transfer may occur at rates of up to 128 Kbps.
ISP	Internet Service Provider. A company that provides its customers access to the Internet and other related services such as e-mail and Web site hosting.
Java	A programming language created by Sun Microsystems, the makers of Applets and JavaScript.
JPEG	One of the two main image formats that are displayed on Web pages. This is excellent for onscreen display of photographs.
Keyboard	The device that permits input into the computer by typing.
Link	A reference to another Web page that can be visited by clicking on the text or graphics that make up the link.
Listserv	A computer program that automatically distributes and redistributes e-mail to names on a mailing list, usually grouped by a similar subject.

Lock-up   A "freeze" of a computer requiring a restart and caus-
                    ing the loss of unsaved information.

Megabyte   A unit of data equal to approximately 1,000,000
                    bytes. On the order of magnitude of the data stored
                    on one $3^1/_2$ inch computer disk.

Microprocessor The brains of the computer; the part that uses simple
                    arithmetic and logic functions to execute complex
                    tasks, such as programs.

Modem   Modulator-demodulator. Device enabling computers
                    to transmit information over telephone lines.

Monitor   The device that displays the computer's functions.

Net   Short for Internet.

.net   A generic suffix for Web pages. Frequently used by
                    individuals or companies that were unable to register
                    their name with the .com suffix.

Netscape   The corporation that created the popular Web browser
                    Navigator.

.org   Short for organization.

PC   Personal computer.

PDA   Personal digital assistant. A hand-held device that
                    performs many of the same functions as a standard-
                    size computer.

pdf   The suffix attached to files that require Adobe Acro-
                    bat for viewing.

Plug in   Software that is complementary and adds special fea-
                    tures to a larger piece of software. This usually is in
                    the form of a plug-in to add effects to a Web browser
                    such as audio or video.

PowerPoint   A program made by Microsoft that creates and dis-
                    plays slide show presentations. The slides may be
                    taken to a photography store for development into
                    plastic slides, or the presentation may be displayed
                    by a special projector directly from the computer.

RAM   Random access memory. The area where the operat-
                    ing system, programs, and data in use are stored so

they can be retrieved rapidly by the microprocessor. The amount of RAM a computer has is often measured in megabytes. The larger the amount of RAM, the quicker the retrieval.

Real audio An example of a plug-in that allows audio and video present on a Web page to be displayed by the visitor's computer.

Search engine Specialized Web page that functions as a topic index for the World Wide Web. It helps you find information online about specific topics.

Server In general, a server is a computer program that provides services to other computer programs. The computer that a server program runs on also is frequently referred to as a server. Specific to the Web, a Web server is the computer program that delivers requested Web pages or files.

Shareware Software distributed free of immediate charge on a trial basis.

Snail mail The old-fashioned way of sending messages. It consists of composing (handwritten or typed) a message, placing it in an envelope, attaching a stamp, and using a postal system for delivery. It often is markedly slower than e-mail, thus the derogatory name.

Software Programs used by computers to accomplish specific tasks.

SPAM Unsolicited electronic mail. The way that these seemingly unrelated terms became synonymous is unclear, but may be based on a Monty Python skit.

Spider A computer program that visits Web pages and records information on them, then reports the information to search engines.

T1 A system that transfers data at 1.544 megabits per second.

T3 A line that allows Internet communication at 44.736 Mbps.

Teleconsultation Use of the Internet to obtain specialist consultation, often in underserved areas.

Telemedicine   Delivery of health care and sharing of medical knowledge using telecommunication systems.

Telementoring   The guidance of a surgeon through a difficult operation by a more experienced surgeon from a distance using the Internet.

Telesurgery   Performing surgery with assistance from the Internet or telemedicine, typically at a significant distance from the patient.

URL   Uniform Resource Locator. This is the "address" where a Web page resides. Its format for Web pages is **http://www. companyname. suffix.country**

User friendly   System that is easy to use, providing help and containing inherently obvious features.

Virus   A contagious piece of program code that causes an unexpected and undesirable event on the recipient's computer.

Web master   Person or persons responsible for production, updates, and administration of a Web page.

Web page   A document, displayed by a browser, that contains text and images and is transferable on the World Wide Web.

WWW   World Wide Web. The portion of the Internet where text, graphics, and sounds are displayed simultaneously with a high degree of user friendliness.

Web   Short for World Wide Web.

Index

Abbot Laboratories, sponsor of Pain Web page, 62

Abdominal masses, pediatric surgery for, 96

Abstracts, online submission of, 74

Access to the Internet, 7–9

Acoustic Neuroma Association, Web site, 93

Acute ischemic stroke, guidelines for patient management, 88

Acute Stroke Toolbox, links page for rapid diagnosis, 88

Address book, for e-mail, 43

Adobe Acrobat, format for Web site newsletter, 71

Adobe Photoshop, to create graphics for Web page, 67

Advanced Research Project Agencies (ARPA), 5–7

Advertising
to pay costs of free e-mail, 41
by physicians on Web pages, 63

Air travel
discounted fares, online, 116
Internet access during, 15

Alta Vista, search engine, 27–28, 118

Amazon.com, 116

American Academy of Neurology, Stroke Coding Guide, 89

American Academy of Orthopaedic Surgeons, Web site, 92

American Academy of Otolaryngology Surgery, Web site, 94

American Association for Hand Surgery, Web site, 84

American Association for the Surgery of Trauma, Web site, 102

American Association for Thoracic Surgery, Web site, 72–73

American Association of Blood Banks, online information from, 73

American Association of Orthopaedic Foot and Ankle Surgeons, Web site, 91–92

American Board of Medical Specialties, 77

American Board of Otolaryngology, Web site, 93–94

American Board of Surgery (ABS), Web site, 77

American Brain Tumor Association, Web site, 88–89

American Cancer Society (ACS), Web site, 78

American College of Sports Medicine (ACSM), Web page, 92

American College of Surgeons, the (ACS), Fellowship of, 79

American Foundation for Urologic Disease, Web site, 81

American Gastroenterological Association, Web site, 75

American Health Consultants, owner of Continuing Medical Education Web site, 61

American Heart Association
guidelines for acute stroke management, 88–89
patient information online, 13
Web site, 73

American Medical Association, study of physician Web pages, 63

American Neurotology Society, Web page, 94–95

American Pediatric Surgical
  Association
  pediatric trauma registry, 104
  Web site, 96
American Red Cross, Web site, 111
American Rhinologic Society, Web
  site, 95
American Society for Aesthetic
  Plastic Surgery (ASAPS), Web
  site, 97–98
American Society for Bariatric
  Surgery, Web site, 70–71
American Society for Surgery of the
  Hand, Web site, 84
American Society of Breast Surgeons,
  Web site, 78
American Society of Colon and
  Rectal Surgeons, Web site, 75
American Society of Plastic
  Surgeons, Web site, 98
American Society of Transplantation,
  Web site, 99
American Trauma Society, Web site,
  102
American Urologic Association
  (AUA), Web site, 81–82
America Online
  e-mail provider, 41
  server space from, 65–66
Anastomotic techniques for surgical
  residents, workshops in, 109
Anatomy
  of the brain, 88
  online pamphlet, 90
  of the hand, with online images, 85
  sinus and nasal, online review of, 95
Anderson, Dr. James, 21
Anesthesia, for plastic surgery, 98
Aneurysm
  aortic, patient information about,
  80
  cranial, online pamphlet about, 90
Aneurysmal subarachnoid
  hemorrhages, guidelines for
  management of, 88

Antiviral software, 22, 24
Apligraf, bioengineered wound care
  product, 107
Appendectomy/appendicitis
  diagnosis of, 96
  patient information about, 80
Apple Computer, 14
Arizona Heart Institute, training
  sessions in vascular surgery,
  109
Armed forces emergency services,
  Red Cross, 111
Arthroscopy
  future use of telesurgery for, 39–40
  and telementoring, 12
Article reader, 19
Association for Morbid Obesity
  Support, Web site, 71
Association of Academic Surgical
  Administrators (AASA), Web
  site, 78
Association of Women Surgeons
  (AWS), Web site, 78–79
Atresia with apple peel deformity,
  pediatric surgery discussion of,
  96
Attachments, to e-mail, 43
Awards, in vascular surgery, 106

Back pain, physician information
  online, 91
Banks, online, 13
Bard Perflix Plug, hernia repair
  system, 107
Bariatric surgery
  Gore Medical products for, 108
  Web resources for, 70–72
Baxter, tissue sealing products, 110
Bellamy, Dr. Ronald, war surgery,
  103
Bicycle injuries, prevention of,
  information online, 104
BioEnterics, Web site, 73
Biomedical services, Red Cross, 111
Bit, defined, 17

Blepharoplasty, patient brochure online, 97
Body mass index, online calculator for, 70–71
Boston Scientific Microinvasive, sponsorship of urology Web site, 82
Bowen, Dr. Thomas E., on war surgery, 103
Brain, anatomy of, 88
  online pamphlet, 91
Brain Tumor Society, Web site, 89
Breast augmentation, patient information about, 98
Brigham and Women's Hospital, digital presentation of uroradiology rounds at, 82–83
Browsers, 1–3
Burn centers, online information about, 97
Byte, defined, 17

Cable News Network, online, 114
Calendar, listing medical conferences and meetings, 61
Callfinder service, for internet telephony, 56
Canadian Association of Pediatric Surgeons, Web page, 96
Cancer
  colorectal, screening and surveillance, 75
  melanoma, 80
  prostate, resource guide online, 81
Cancer-specific Web pages, 78
Cardiac and thoracic surgery, 72–75
Cardiac blunt injury, management guidelines, 102
Cardiology, and telemedicine, 37
Cardiopulmonary bypass, tissue adhesives used in, 110
Cardiothoracic products, Gore Medical, 108
Cardiothoracic Surgery Network, Web site, 74

Carotid shunts, 109
Carpal tunnel syndrome, neurosurgery, resource page online, 91
Cataloging, of material on the Web, 31–32
"Caveat viewor", regarding accuracy of information, 21
Cellular phone, use with laptop computer, 15
Centers for Disease Control, Web site, 103–104, 111
Center Watch, online resource about clinical studies, 34
Chat rooms, 12, 24, 52–53
Chatting online, 52–57
  with experts on facial neuralgia, 90
  for urologists, 82
Chemical peel, patient information about, 98
Chemotherapy, treatment for brain tumors, 89
Chiari malformation, online pamphlet about, 91
Childhood ailments, common, diagnosis of, 97
Chittmittrapap, Professor Soottiporn, pediatric surgery images, 97
Cholocystectomy, laparoscopic patient information about, 80
  use of harmonic scalpel in, 108
Chulalongkorn University Hospital (Thailand), pediatric surgery at, 97
Cinema, Web sites for, 115
Clinical trials
  data from, on brain tumors, 89
  information about, National Institutes of Health, 34–35
  information from a cardiac Web site, 74
  references to, on World Wide Web, 11
  of surgical treatment for brain tumors, 89

Clinical Trials, Web page, National
Institutes of Health, 112
Clinical Trials and Noteworthy
Treatments for Brain Tumors,
Web page, 89
Clinical Trials Resource Center,
online information about clinical
studies, 34
CME Web, Web resource offering
courses, 61
Coagulation disorders, links specific
to, 105
Cochlear implants, essays online, 93
Coding and reimbursement, for
orthopaedic procedures, 91–92
Colon
injuries to, penetrating
intraperitoneal, 102
resection of, use of harmonic
scalpel in, 108
Colonoscopy, patient information
about, 80
Colorectal Cancer Screening, Web
page, 75
Colorectal surgery, Web resources
about, 75–77
Colostomy closure, tissue adhesives
for, 110
Commercial use of the Internet, 7
Compact disc read only memory
(CD-ROM), 16, 23
Complication management, and
telesurgery, 39
Composix, for ventral hernia repair, 107
Computed tomography (CT) scans
in answers to sample questions, 79
in uroradiology rounds, online, 82
Computer crashes, avoiding, 22–23
Computer freeze, 22
Computer genre, Apple and
International Business Machines,
14
Concussion, physician information
online, 91

Connection rate, of an Internet
service provider, 17
Consensus Development Conference
on Gastrointestinal Surgery for
Severe Obesity, NIH Statement
online, 72
Contemporary Urology, Web site, 82
Continuing medical education (CME),
58–62
about lymphatic mapping, 109
Medline courses online, 113
programs in otolaryngology, 93–94
about sentinel lymph node biopsy,
110
in trauma surgery, 102
in vascular surgery, 109
on the World Wide Web, 11
Cook, surgical products Web site, 107
Cost
of domain hosting, 65
of Web page design, 64
Country suffix, 3
Credit cards
online use of, 13
use to pay for Continuing Medical
Education, 61
Crohn's and Colitis Foundation of
America
patient information online, 13
Web site, 76
Crohn's disease, patient information,
113
Cyberpatrol, 24
Cyber Sitter, 24

Data identification (ID), to encrypt
files for transfer, 51
DeBakey, Dr. Michael, use of the
Internet to follow patients, 38
Defense Advanced Research Projects
Agency (DARPA), 6–7
Department of Health and Human
Services, organ donation
resources, 100

Dermabound, topical skin adhesive, 108

Dermatology, and telemedicine, 37

Design, professional, of Web pages, 64

Desktop computer versus laptop, 15–16

Dialpad, Internet telephony, 56

Dialysis unit personnel, workshops for, 109

Digestive Disease Week, conference information, 76

Digital Urology Journal, online peer-reviewed journal, 82–83

Digital video disc (DVD), 16

Disaster services, Red Cross, 111

Diverticulitis, surgical management of, 76

Domain hosting services, 65

Domain Name System, 7

Domains
  international suffixes, 125–128
  top level, common, 129
  See also Suffixes

Domestic violence, prevention of, information online, 103–104

Downloading files, 23–24

Dr. Koop, Web site, 112

Drugs
  for cancer, information about, 78
  interactions among, new and under development, 113
  for malaria, 111
  online reference guide, 19
  pharmacology of therapy using, associated with surgery, 81
  prescription, online availability of, 13

Early diagnosis examples, on physician Web pages, 63

Eastern Association for Surgery of Trauma, Web page, 102

E-commerce, 13

E-Hand, Electronic Handbook of Hand Surgery, Web site, 84–85

Electrocardiogram, as an e-mail attachment, 43

Electronic mail (e-mail), 4, 11–12, 41–51
  lists for exchanging information, 53
  ten commandments for communicating with patients, 45
  viruses attached to, 23

Emergency War Surgery, handbook online, 103

Encryption, of patients records, 51

Endoscopy
  future use of telesurgery for, 39–40
  and telemedicine, 37
  and telementoring, 12

Epilepsy, neurosurgery, resource page online, 91

EPocrates, drug reference guide, 19

Erectile dysfunction, reviews online, 82

Ethicon, surgical products Web site, 108

Eudora
  e-mail software, 43
  Secure Multi-Process Internet Mail Extensions of, 51

European Association for Endoscopic Surgery (EAES), Web site, 86

European Society for Vascular Surgery, Web page, 105

Ewing's sarcoma, chat rooms about, 53

Examinations, offered by the American Board of Surgery, 77

Eyelid surgery, patient information about, 98

Eye problems, following acoustic neuroma surgery, 93

Face Book, The, from an online bookstore, 97

Facial Neuralgia Resources, Web
    page, 89–90
Facial weakness or paralysis, following
    acoustic neuroma surgery, 93
Favretti, Dr. Franco, laparoscopic
    telesurgery, 39
Federal Trade Commission (FTC),
    role in assuring accuracy of Web
    sites, 21
Fee schedule, for teleconsultation, 38
Fellowships
    in critical care medicine, 104
    in hand surgery, 84–85
    information about, online, 73
    in trauma surgery, 102
Female urology, reviews online, 82
Fetal monitoring, interactive, 37
Fiberoptic devices, online information
    for BioEnterics, 72
Fibrin tissue adhesives, for surgical
    healing and hemostasis, 110
File Transfer Protocol (FTP), 4
    for moving files to a server, 65, 67
Filo, David, 29
Filters, avoiding unwanted
    information with, 24–25
Floppy disk drive, 16
Floppy disks, backing up to, 23
Food and Drug Administration
    (FDA), approval of LAP-BAND,
    anticipated, 72
Forehead lifts, patient brochure
    online, 97
Frequently asked questions (FAQ)
    brain tumors, 89
    on physician Web pages, 63
    about renal transplants, 100
Fundoplication, use of harmonic
    scalpel in, 108

Gamma-ray guided surgery,
    technologies for, Neoprobe, 109
Gastrointestinal bleeding
    and pediatric surgery, 97
    when to refer to a specialist, 80

Gastrostomy, products for, Moss
    Tubes, 109
General medicine, 111–113
General public, medical information
    for, 113
General Surgery, Web resources
    about, 77–80
General Surgery Patient Information,
    links page, 80
Genitourinary surgery, Web resources
    for, 81–84
Genzyme Surgical Products
    sponsor of Heart Surgery Forum,
    74
    Web site, 108
Geographic specific health threats,
    information online, 111
G.G.'s Dignity Wear Inc., sponsor of
    online information for ostomy
    patients, 76–77
Gibbon, John H. Jr., Research
    Scholarship, 73
Gigabyte (Gb), defined, 17
Glasgow Coma Score, outline, online,
    102
Glioblastoma, chat rooms about,
    53
Glitches, in computers, 22–23
Glossary, 131-135
Glucose control, interactive, 37
Go2Call, for Internet telephony, 56
Google, search engine, 28
Gore, W.L. & Associates, a sponsor
    of the Journal of Vascular
    Surgery, 105
Gore Medical, surgical products, Web
    site, 108
Graffiti writing system, 19
Grafts, polyester, 109
Grants. See Fellowships; Research
    awards; Scholarships
Graphics, for attachment to e-mail,
    43
Gynecologic surgical products, Gore
    Medical, 109

Hair replacements, patient brochure online, 97

Hand surgery, Web resources about, 84–86

Hand Transplant, Web site, 85

Hard copy, defined, 16

Hard drive, 16

Hardware, needed for accessing the Internet, 14–18

Harmonic Scalpel, Web site, 108

Harvard Medical School, pediatric uroradiology rounds at, 83

Head injuries, neurosurgery for, resource page online, 91

HealthAtoZ Professional, affiliation with MedConnect, 62

Health Care Learning and Information Exchange (HELIX), Continuing Medical Education resource, 58–62

Healtheon, Web site, 113

Healthgate
database, 35–36
Web page, 113

Health Insurance Portability and Accountability Act (HIPPA), transfer of patient medical records under, 50–51

Health maintenance organizations (HMO), Internet guide to, 96

Health-related Internet resources, 111–118

Health-related Web sites, scientific validity of, 20

Health Resources and Services Administration, organ donation resources, 100

Hearing aid, essay on purchasing, 93

Hearing Education and Awareness for Rockers (H.E.A.R.), Web page, 95

Hearing loss, following acoustic neuroma surgery, 93

Heart
diseases of, online information about, 73
minimally invasive direct coronary artery bypass, e-mail forum about, 74
mitral valve replacement, Internet for following patients, 38
transplantation of, statistics online, 100

Heart Surgery Forum, Web site, 74

Hemorrhoids, patient information, 113

Hemostasis, clinical aspects of, online, 105

Heparin-associated thrombocytopenia, pathophysiology of, online, 105

Herniated disks, neurosurgery, resource page online, 91

Hirschprung's disease, diagnosis of, 96

Historical record
antique illnesses, interactive Web site on diagnosis, 80
William P. Didusch Museum, 81–82

Home page, defined, 3

Hot Bot, search engine, 29

Hotel rooms, reserving online, 116

Hotmail, e-mail provider, 41

Hydrocephalus Association, Web site, 90–91

Hypertext Mark-up Language (HTML), 1
for creating a Web page, 66
flexibility for Continuing Medical Education modules, 59

Hypertext Transfer Protocol (HTTP), 1–3

ICQ, software for online chats, 53

Immunizations, suggested, 111

Immunotherapy, treatment for brain tumors, 89

Impra, products for vascular surgery, 109

Inflammatory bowel disease, online information about, 76

Information, finding, 26–32

Injury. *See* Trauma

Instant messages, 54

Integrated Services Digital Network (ISDN), connection to the Internet via, 17–18

International Business Machines (IBM), 14

International Federation for the Surgery of Obesity, Web site, 72

International Hand Library, Web site, 86

International Museum of Surgical Science, Web site, 80

International Society for Computer Aided Surgery, Web site, 86

International Society for Heart and Lung Transplant, Web site, 100

International Society for Minimally Invasive Cardiac Surgery, Web site, 74

Internet
   advantages for Continuing Medical Education, 58–59
   connecting to, 14–19
   defined, 7
   described, 1–3
   history of, 2–9
   speed of connections, 16–18

Internet Content Rating Association, 24

Internet for Physicians, The (Smith), 11

Internet hub, 9

Internet Movie Database, 116

Internet Service Provider (ISP), 12, 14, 16, 41
   server space provided by, 65

Internet telephony, 55–57

Interventional Laparoscopy: The State of the Art . . . , excerpts online, 87

Intragastric balloon system, 72

Intravenous pylograms, uroradiology rounds, online, 83

Investing, Web sites for, 117

Jasc Paintshop Pro, to create graphics for Web page, 67

Jejunostomy, products for, Moss Tubes, 109

Job information
   from the American College of Surgeons, 79
   from a cardiac Web site, 74
   in critical care medicine, 104
   from Digestive Disease Week, 76
   internship opportunities in surgery, 78
   at Stryker Instruments, 110
   in transplant surgery, 99
   in trauma surgery, 102

Johnson & Johnson, harmonic scalpel, 108

Journal of GI Surgery, links to an online version, 76

Journal of Pediatric Laparoscopy, online, 87

Journal of the Society of Laparoendoscopic Surgeons, Web site under construction, 88

Journal of Thoracic and Cardiovascular Surgery, Web site, 72–73

Journal of Vascular Surgery, Web page, 105

Journals, *Digital Urology Journal*, 82–83. *See also* specific *Journal of . . .* entries

Karl Storz, endoscopy equipment, Web site, 109

Keyboard, 16
   of personal digital assistants, 19

Kilobit (Kb), defined, 17

Kleinrock, Leonard, 6

Koop, Dr. C. Everett, 112

Laetrile, advertised on web, 21
Laparoscopic gastric band
    LAP-BAND adjustable gastric
        banding system, 72
    telesurgery for, at a short distance,
        39
Laparoscopy
    future use of telesurgery for, 39–40
    instruments for, 108
    pediatric surgery, 97
    and telementoring, 12
    training in, using telementoring, 40
    using robots and the Internet, 39
Laparoscopy.com, Web site, 86
Laparoscopy.net, Web site, 87
Laptop computer versus desktop,
    15–16
Levinson, Dr. Mark, 74
Libraries, Internet hub offered by, 9
Licensing issues, and telesurgery, 39
Licklider, J.C.R., 6
LifeLine Foundation, promotion and
    funding, 106
Linking process, 2
Lipoinfo, Web site, 98
Liposuction, patient information
    about, 98
Literature searches, 11, 35–37
Local area networks (LANs), 7
Lung transplant, statistics online, 100
Lycos, 118
    news pages, 115

Macintosh operating system, 10–11
Magnetic resonance images,
    uroradiology rounds, online, 83
Majure, Dr. Joyce A., 78
Malarone, antimalarial drug, 111
Maps and directions
    online, 117
    on physician Web pages, 63
Massachusetts Institute of Technology
    (MIT), 6
MedConnect, Continuing Medical
    Education center, 62

Medical applications, of e-mail,
    guidelines for, 44–50
Medical calculator, 19
Medical information, on the Internet,
    20–25
Medical records, electronic transfer
    of, 51
MEDLINE database
    literature searches, 35–36
    physician database, link to, 106
    searching, 113
    search of citations from, 113
MedPortal database, 35–36
Medscape
    Continuing Medical Education
        center, 59–61
    database, 35–36
    drug reference guide, 19
    as an e-mail provider, 41
    Web page templates from,
        67–68
    Web site, 113
Megabyte (MB), defined, 17
Melanoma, when to refer to a
    specialist, 80
Microprocessor, 16
    computer, 18
Microsoft browser, Secure Multi-
    Process Internet Mail Extensions
    of, 51
Microsoft Internet Explorer, 3, 41
Microsoft Outlook Express, 41–43
Microsoft Paint, to create graphics for
    Web page, 67
Microsoft Windows, 10, 14
    initial release of, 7
Microsoft Word
    documents online, 93–94
    using to create HTML files, 66
Minimal access surgery, Web
    resources for, 87. *See also*
    Laparoscopy
Minimally invasive direct coronary
    artery bypass (MIDCAB), e-mail
    forum about, 74

Mitral valve replacement, use of the Internet to follow patients following, 38

Modem (modulator demodulator), 10–11, 16
cable, 18
for Internet access, 15
speed of, 17

Money Magazine, online, 117

Monitor, 16

Morbid obesity, surgery for treating, 70–72

Moss Tubes, products for gastrostomy, 109

Motor vehicle accidents, prevention of, information online, 103–104

Mouse, 16

Moving Picture Expert Group-1, Audio Layer-3 (MP3), music format, 115

Multiple myeloma, chat room for, 53

Munchausen syndrome
in chat rooms, 53
online, 24

Musella Foundation for Brain Tumor Research, Web site, 89

Music, Web sites for, 115

Myringotomy tubes, when to refer to a specialist, 80

Nasal endoscopy, introduction to, online, 95

National Aeronautics and Space Administration (NASA), 5

National Association for Biomedical Research, online information from, 73

National Center for Injury Prevention and Control, Web page, 103–104

National Institute of Disability and Rehabilitation Research, pediatric trauma registry, 103–104

National Institutes of Health (NIH) clinical trials Web page, 112

online information about clinical studies, 34
Web site, 72

National Language Searching (NLS), 37

National Library of Medicine
clinical trials Web page, 112
PubMed search service, 113

National Pediatric Trauma Registry, Web page, 104

National Science Foundation, 7

Navy, U.S.
surgical telementoring aboard the U.S.S. Abraham Lincoln, 40
Virtual Naval Hospital, 103

Neoprobe, sentinel lymph node technologies, 109

Netscape
browser, Secure Multi-Process Internet Mail Extensions of, 51
news pages, 115

Netscape Navigator, 3, 41

Network Control Protocol, 6

Networks, dedicated, for telemedicine, 37

Neurosurgery
traumatic, triage with telemedicine, 38
Web resources for, 88–91

Neurosurgery on Call, Web page, 91

Neurosurgical Focus, online peer-reviewed journal, 92

New England Medical Center, pediatric trauma registry, 104

News, Web sites for, 115

Nontraditional medical services, advertising on the Web, 21

Novartis Pharmaceuticals Corporation, wound care products, 107

Obesity, Web sites about, 70–72

Office hours, listing on physician Web pages, 63

Oncology, reviews online, 82

Order, of topical lists, search engines, 31

Organ Donation, Web site, 100

Organ injuries, guidelines for grading, online, 102

Orthopedic surgery, Web resources for, 92

Otolaryngologic Surgery, Web resources for, 93–96

Otolaryngology Training Examination (OTE), coverage online, 93–94

Outlook Express, Secure Multi-Process Internet Mail Extensions of, 51

Ouzounian, Dr. Tye, on coding procedures, 91–92

Packet switching, 5–6
  Domain Name System, 7

Page Rank, technology used in Google, 29

Pain, Web page for, Continuing Medical Education modules, 62

Pain pump, Stryker Instruments, 110

Palm Pilot, 118
  personal digital assistant, 44

Pathology, and telemedicine, 37

Patient accrual, for clinical trials, 33

Patient data, transmitting by e-mail, 51

Patient follow-up, using the Internet for, 38

Patient information
  about brain tumors, 88–89
  about cancer, 78
  about cleft lips or palates, 96
  about colorectal surgery, 75
  about Crohn's disease and colitis, 76
  health news and medical information, 113
  about hydrocephalus, 90
  about neurosurgery, 91
  about otolaryngology surgery, 93

about overactive bladders and incontinence, 81
about plastic and reconstructive surgery, 98
about plastic surgery, 98–99
about renal transplantation, 100
about surgery, 80
about surgical procedures, 79
about thoracic surgery, 75
on Web pages, misguided, 20–21
on the World Wide Web, 11

Pediatric Burns, Web site, 97

Pediatric Laparoscopy, Web site, 87

Pediatric surgery, Web resources for, 96–98

Pediatric trauma, guidelines for managing, online, 104

Personal digital assistant (PDA), 18–19, 44

Personal home page, physician's, 13

Personal Web page
  through Medscape, 113
  for orthopedic surgeons, 91
  saving addresses on, 21

Photographs
  images of traumatic injuries, 104
  intraoperative
  hand transplant, 85
  of pediatric surgery, 96

Physician recruitment, via the Internet, 33

Physician Resources, in Neurosurgery on Call, 91

Physicians Online, Web site, 113

Pierre Robin syndrome, information about, online, 96

Pitfalls, in patient communication using e-mail, 46–50

Plastic and reconstructive surgery, Web resources for, 97–98

Plastic Surgery Educational Foundation
  Web page, 98

Plastic Surgery Information Services, Web page, 98

Pocket Mentor (Majure), manual for surgical interns, 78–79

Polypropylene, polytetrafluoroethylene (PTFE), for a ventral hernia repair mesh, 107

Pornography, online, 24–25

Postoperative conditions, information on physician Web pages, 63

Power Point format, inclusion in Web sites, 74

Prescription medicines, online availability of, 13

Prescription refill directions, on physician Web pages, 63

Primary care physician
  guidelines for surgical management, 76
  guide to brain tumors for, 89

Prisoners, medical care of, and telemedicine, 38

Product surveys online, in urology, compensated, 81

Protocols, for the Internet, 7

PubMed
  database, 35–36
  search service, 113

Quality Surgical Solutions, Web site, 80

Quilici, Dr. Philippe J., 87

Radiation, for brain tumors, 89

Radiographs
  digital images of, 12
  of the hand, online images, 85
  high-definition, as an e-mail attachment, 43
  images from pediatric surgery, 97
  of traumatic injuries, 104
  uroradiology rounds, online, 82
  See also Photographs

Radio-guided parathyroidectomy, patient information about, 80

Radiology, and telemedicine, 37

Random access memory (RAM), 16, 18

Real Audio player, 114
  format on Web sites, 74
  used on a surgical Web site, 79

Reconstructive surgery, cleft lips and palates, 96

Referrals, online, for laparoscopic surgery, 86–87

Rehabilitation, in acoustic neuroma, 93

Renal transplantation, patient information about, 100

Rental cars, reserving online, 116

Research and Training Center in Rehabilitation and Childhood Trauma, registry, 104

Research awards
  in brain tumors, 89
  in hand surgery, 84
  in hydrocephalus, 90
  in rhinology, 95
  in thoracic surgery, 75
  in vascular surgery, 106
  See also Fellowships; Scholarships

Resistance, to the Internet, 10

Rhinoplasty, patient brochure online, 97

Rhône-Poulenc-Rorer, sponsor of brain tumor Web site, 89

RIGS technique, from Neoprobe, 109

Robert Wood Johnson Medical School, host for pediatric surgery site, 96

St. Joseph's Medical Center, Burbank, California, laparoscopy Web page, 87

Scar revision, patient brochure online, 97

Scholarships
  information about, online, 73
  in neurotology, 94
  in pediatric urology, 82
  in thoracic surgery, 75

for work related to hydrocephalus, 90

Scientific American Medicine, online version, 113

Scott, Matthew, first hand transplant patient, 85

Search engines, 27–32

Searching
creating a phrase for, 36–37
tips for, 30–31

Seldinger, Sven-Ivan, Cook medical group, 107

Sentinel lymph node biopsy, guidelines for, 78

Seprafilm, to decrease postoperative adhesions, 107

Sepramesh, for postoperative wounds, 108

Servers, getting Web page information to, 65

Shaken baby syndrome, physician information online, 91

Short bowel syndrome, study of, protocols and consent forms, 96

Silicone devices, online information from BioEnterics, 72

Sinus and nasal anatomy, overview online, 95

Skin adhesive, topical, 108

Skin construct, bilayered viable, 107

S/MIME (Secure Multi-Process Internet Mail Extensions), for sending encrypted e-mail, 51

Society for Pediatric Urology, Web site, 83

Society for Surgery of the Alimentary Tract, Web site, 76

Society of American Gastrointestinal Endoscopic Surgeons, Web site, 87

Society of Critical Care Medicine, Web site, 104

Society of Laparoendoscopic Surgeons (SLS), Web site, 88

Society of Thoracic Surgeons, Web site, 74–75

Soft tissue hand injuries, description online, 84

Software
antiviral, 24
Eudora, for e-mail software, 43
Microsoft Internet Explorer, 41
Microsoft Outlook Express, 41–43
Netscape Navigator, 41
for online chats, NetMeeting, 55
for using "Online Surgery", 79

Sound card, 16

Soviet Union, fear of, 6

SPAM, 43–44

Spiders, assembling search engine database, 32

Spinal leak, following acoustic neuroma surgery, 93

Sports, injuries related to, physician information online, 92

Sports Illustrated, Web page, 114

Sputnik, 5

Stock market, Web sites for, 117

Stroke
neurosurgery in, resource page online, 91
online information about, 73

Stroke Coding Guide, of the American Academy of Neurology, online, 88

Stryker Instruments, products for surgical procedures, 110

Suffixes
.com, 3
.edu, 3
.gif, 67
.gov, 3
.jpeg, 67
See also Domains

Suicide, prevention of, information online, 104

Sunbelt Melanoma Trial, Web page of, 35

Support for People with Oral and
  Head and Neck Cancer
  patient information online, 13
  Web page, 95
Support groups, online, use of chat
  rooms, 53
Surfing, advanced, 18–19, 36–37,
  50–51
Surf Watch, 24
Surgeon certification status, online
  inquiries about, 77
Surgery
  archived procedures, online, 79
  general, products online, 107–110
  techniques for, in emergency war
    surgery, 103
  Web pages for departments of,
    United States by state, 119–124
Surgical Education Self-Assessment
  Program (SESAP), sample
  radiographs, high definition, 79
Surgical Endoscopy, links to, 86
Surgical practices
  using e-mail in, 44
  Web pages for specialties, 70–110
Suture, braided synthetic absorbable,
  108

T1 and T3 connections, 18
Teleconsulting, 38
Telemedicine, 12–13, 37–40
  information about clinical trials,
    33–35
Telementoring, 12–13, 39
Teleradiology, 12, 38
Telesurgery, 38–39
Template, to create Web pages,
  67–68
Tertiary care centers, telemedicine for
  routing patients to, 38
Testicular torsion, diagnosis of, 98
Thermonuclear war, trauma surgery
  in, 103
Third ventriculostomy, description
  online, 90–91

Thoracic Surgery Foundation for
  Research and Education, Web
  site, 75
Thoracoscopy, and telementoring, 12
Thrombolytic therapy, for acute
  stroke, links to guidelines for,
  88
Thrombosis, clinical aspects of,
  online, 106
Thrombosite, Web page, 105
Tinnitus
  following acoustic neuroma
    surgery, 93
  information online, 95
Tissue Sealing, Web site, 110
Top level domains, 3
Training, in laparoscopy, using
  telementoring, 40
Transmission Control
  Protocol/Internet Protocol
  (TCP/IP), 7
Transplant Awareness, Inc., Web site,
  100
Transplant Patient Partnering, Web
  page, 100
Transplant surgery, Web resources
  for, 99–101
Transweb, Web site, 101
Trauma
  information about courses, online,
    102
  prevention of, information online,
    102
  surgical treatment of, Web
    resources for, 102–104
  vascular, clinical strategies and
    current opinion, 105
Trauma.org, Web site, 104
Traumatic splenetic injuries, tissue
  adhesives for, 110
Travel, Web sites for, 116
Traveler's Health, Web site, Centers
  for Disease Control, 111
Triage, telemedicine for, 38
Trigemial Neuralgia Association

International Conference (1998), report available online, 90
Truman, President Harry S, on persecution of American scientists, 5
Tumors
of the brain, 89
Ewing's sarcoma chat rooms, 53
malignant, head and neck, 95
Tuvalu, sale of domain name, 129

Ulcerative colitis, online information about, 76
Uniform Resource Locator (URL), 26 components of, 2–3
United Ostomy Association, Web site, 76–77
United States Federal Networking Council, defined, 7
University Children's Hospital (Zurich), pediatric burn information online, 97
University of Chicago, training sessions in vascular surgery, 109
University of the Sciences (Philadelphia), affiliation with MedConnect, 62
University of Washington Continuing Medical Education resource, 62
Urology, pediatric, reviews online, 82
Urology News, Web site, bimonthly review, 83
Uronet
Web page, 84
Uroreviews, Web page, 84
User friendly context, development of, 10–11

Validity, of information from health related Web sites, 20
Vargas, Dr. Miguel, hand therapist award, 84
Vascular and endovascular grafts, 109
Vascular probes, 109

Vascular Surgeries Societies Homepage, Web site, 106
Vascular surgery, Web resources for, 105–106
Vendor marketplace, hand surgery-related, 86
Video conferencing, in chat rooms, 11–12
Video images, in laparoscopy, 86–87
Video signal, integration into chatting, 55
Virtual Naval Hospital, war surgery handbook, 103
Viruses, computer, 22–24
Voice conference, using Yahoo! Messenger, 54–55
Volunteering, Red Cross, 111

Waiting lists, discussion about, for transplants, 101
Wall Street Journal, online, 117
Wand, data entry with, 19
Web-based Injury Statistics Query and Reporting System (WISQUARS), 104
Web browsers, for sending encrypted e-mail, 51
WebMD
Web page templates from, 67–68
Web site, 113
Web pages, 2–3
homemade, 66–67
illegal, contraband music on, 115
inclusion in search engines, 32
nonmedical, 114–118
patient information from, validity of, 20–21
for physicians, 63–110
production of, 64
viewing, 26–27
Web site, defined, 3
Wide Smiles, Cleft Lip, and Palate Resource, Web site, 96
Wire, The, news pages, 115
Wireless Internet access, 19

Wisconsin, University of, 7
WordPerfect (Corel), documents
    online, 93
World Congress of Minimally
    Invasive Cardiac Surgery, 74
World of Pediatric Surgery, Web site,
    97
World Wide Web (WWW), 1–3,
    9–11, 14
  for Continuing Medical Education
    in surgery, 58
  disease-specific information on, 53
  indexing by search engines, 27
  maps and directions for travel, 117
  music sources on, 115

for searching the medical literature,
    35–36
Wound care products, Web resources
    for identifying, 107
Wound profiles, for a M-16 weapon,
    103

Yahoo!
  e-mail provider, 41
  search engine, 29
  tracking personal interests with,
    118
Yahoo! Messenger, software for
    online chats, 54–55
Yang, Jerry, 29